A LIFE *Worth* LIVING

One woman's story of living with cancer through love, support, and faith.

Written by
MIMI DEETHS

Compiled by
ELIZABETH DEETHS

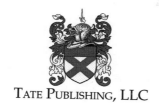

TATE PUBLISHING, LLC

Note

Mimi was a great writer who loved the Lord.

Several of her entries are in journal format, some are actual speeches, and others are letters of love penned for her family and friends.

If Mimi wasn't your friend, then it was because you hadn't met. Her heart continues throughout eternity through the words she has written. Some entries have been lightly edited; others have been left intact to reflect Mimi's thoughts and feelings.

This is an honest look at a "mean disease" through the eyes and heart and soul of a kind woman who understood true love. Some people travel their entire life's journey and never live; Mimi lived her entire life as she traveled her journey.

Acknowledgements

I would like to dedicate this book to my mom, Mary Catherine (Davy) Deeths, known to all by Mimi. I strive to be like her as I go through life. She was a wife, a mother, a daughter, and a friend to all. She touched countless people's lives. Through this book, she will continue to touch lives for years to come. She will never be forgotten. I love you, Mom and I miss you. May this book be a tribute to your life.

And to my family. M.J., Dad, Christine, Katie, Jeff, David, and Timothy, this book is for you. You have your memories, but now you have her words as well.

I would like to give a special thanks to Brad and Cindy Webb, Mary Richard, Marcia Monsma, Jennifer Black, Betty Serati, Nancy Pelton, Triss Meyer, Amparo Kinnsch, Debbie Davis, Ravi Patel and Homer, Kevin, and Kendon Kuo. Thank you for sharing your thoughts on my mom. I know I gave you a difficult assignment, so thank you.

To Mary Richard and Iva Davison, who were among the few who knew of my "secret project." I needed someone to share my excitement with and to give me advice. Thank you for keeping my secret.

To all of Mimi's family and friends. She loved you all, thank you for being a part of her life.

To all the doctor's and nurses who treated my Mom. She was always treated with respect and dignity. She befriended many of you. Thank you.

To all those at Tate Publishing. Thank you for investing in this book and believing in my mom's story and the impact it can have on others.

And to God . . . all things are possible through You.

Elizabeth Deeths
alifeworthliving2004@yahoo.com

Foreword

by
Ravi Patel, M.D.

As cancer professionals, we come across people who ask, "Why have you chosen the profession of oncology? Isn't it a depressing and discouraging field? Would you choose this profession again if you had a chance to do so?"

My answer to this is a clear yes.

This is because of the fact that as an oncologist you have an opportunity to come into the lives of patients with cancer when they need you the most. This relationship often becomes a spiritual journey where the patient will not only transform your life but also the lives of others they come in contact with. Mimi Deeths was such a person. Knowing her and caring for her became a lesson in personal growth. Knowing her gave you the understanding that the diagnosis of cancer, or any bad situation in life, can be depressing or discouraging only if you choose to allow it to be that way.

As an example, often breaking the news of the diagnosis of cancer to a patient is difficult both for the patient and the physician. I was wondering how was I going to tell this young individual of 45 with such a loving family that she had metastatic cancer to the liver, and that we would need to give her chemotherapy with all the side effects involving the same. But Mimi made the whole process easier and comfortable for me, as well as all the other members of her family.

The first meeting itself revealed the true nature of Mimi and her openness and willingness to always accept whatever came along. She was in her room with her family, laughing and joking in the hospital, celebrating her birthday with everyone wearing pig noses and eating chocolate cake a few days after her surgery when I went by to visit her for the first time. I remember sitting down and explaining to Mimi the findings of her cancer involving the liver, the need for further testing, and the need for chemotherapy. Even with such disappointing news, it was amazing to see what a beautiful attitude she had. Instead of people around her providing her with support to deal with her illness, her own attitude and behavior strengthened and encouraged the people who were around her, including myself.

From then onwards began a 10-year period of continued treatment of some kind or another; she was either getting chemotherapy or radiation therapy or surgery. At the prime of her life, she had to go through numerous "disappointing events," but for Mimi, these were not disappointing events at all. She moved through them all with amazing grace and beauty. Many people with the amount of treatments and disappointments that Mimi went though would become embittered about life in general and become difficult to deal with.

But in Mimi's situation, it was exactly the opposite. The more she was challenged by these events, the greater the reflection of her inner strength and beauty. There was always acceptance and surrender to God, no matter how things unfolded. This was one of the most beautiful things to see in her. There was never a feeling of "Why me? Why do I need to go through this? This treatment is terrible." Even when she was hospitalized for severe side effects of the treatment, there were no complaints, just this "gentle will" to do what needed to be done and to take the next step forward in continuing her life for her family, friends, and church.

Even when her disease advanced, Mimi would always be patient. There were many days when I would be delayed by emergencies, and Mimi would sit patiently for 45 minutes to an hour waiting to see me. But in spite of this, in all the years we cared for Mimi, there was never a day when there was any anger or resentment on keeping her waiting. Even though Mimi waited for such long periods of time for her visits, she was so kind that she wrote numerous notes of how appreciative she was for me seeing her. Little did she know that I appreciated her coming into my life and the lives of so many other people.

It was a joy to see her at every visit. She always had a smile and always had questions about how other people were doing. She was like the shining light of a flawless diamond with the softness and gentleness of a beautiful flower. Just like a flawless diamond, she had no flaws in her character. I cannot recall in her any negative quality. She was always gentle, kind, giving and inspiring. She made it a point to go out of her way in lifting the spirits of all the people she came in contact with even though she herself was suffering. I often have thought, when I've thought of Mimi, how open she was in welcoming everybody and every situation that came into her life. She rejected nothing. She was always an inspiration for other patients, the nurses and the staff, and their children. She touched the lives of so many in such a way that it was not surprising to see tears roll down the cheeks of many who thought of her.

A few years ago, we had our first Celebration of Life with the opening of a universal chapel. This was followed again by a second Celebration of Life. During both these events, Mimi was going through pretty aggressive treatment and was quite weak, but yet she would sacrifice her own discomforts and showed up at these Celebrations of Life just so that other people would be able to enjoy her presence. It is because of people like Mimi that this "medical profession" becomes a spiritual journey. This is why I would not change my profession.

There is an old Hindu saying that states "The whole world is my family."

Mimi was a living example of this. To her, the whole world truly was her family. It was not "How can others help me?" but "Even with everything that is happening in my life, what can I do to make the lives of others better?" As an oncologist, I wonder why people have to suffer? Why do they need to go through so many disappointments? Why do people have to die so young given that they mean so much to others? I don't think we have the answers to these questions, but it is because you come to know patients like Mimi that the search for these questions becomes meaningful. I hope each of you who read this get a chance in your lifetime to meet a shining star such as Mimi Deeths.

A sincere thanks to the wonderful Deeths family for making me part of this.

Ravi Patel, M.D.
Comprehensive Blood and Cancer Center, Bakersfield, CA

Foreword

By
Tony Deeths & Family
2/13/04

As I read all the Christmas cards and letters this year, I was struck by guilt at not writing my own letter for several years. We have so many friends, and yet I have not done my part in keeping them a part of our lives. As Mimi's illness progressed over the last three years, I have not had the heart to write my usual letter, but mostly, Mimi would not send a letter without rereading your letters and including a personal note for each of you. As the cancer progressed, she just didn't have the stamina for such a large task, but I know that she did still keep contact with many of you by cards and calls.

On February 6, 2004 she ultimately defeated her cancer and returned to her God. Such was the love of her children that they were all home for her last several weeks—caring for her bodily needs–comforting her–lying with her—holding her as she died—dressing her in her 'Mother of the Bride' dress for her last trip out of the house.

All of you know her in different ways: her school friends as a young lady with dreams of a career, a young doctor and a family, her St. Louis friends as a young mother devoted to her children's education and welfare, her Bakersfield friends as someone who would rather do for others than dwell on her cancer and the constant physical and mental burden it imposed. The one common memory, however, was her loving and caring nature.

Most of you are unaware of how profound her illnesses were. She had scoliosis as a child, and about fifteen years ago due to child-bearing and child carrying, the pain and curve started to become progressively worse. Never one to complain, she would gut it out without medication. After the move to Bakersfield, however, things had reached the point where she could not control the pain, and she was becoming deformed from the curve. Twelve years ago she had surgery and began a one and a half year recovery in a back brace.

In June of 1994, at the age of 45, she was preparing to visit Chicago for the annual lake party. She had been experiencing GI problems for several months, but in her usual fashion, she minimized her physical problems. Finally, she submitted to a colonoscopy and a large tumor was discovered. We arranged for surgery the next day. The news was devastating—a large tumor of the colon with local extension and nodes and diffuse metastatic involvement of the liver. Her two-year survival probability was less than 2%. The day after surgery was her birthday. By then, the kids had all arrived; to distract them, I sent them out for party decorations. In a pattern that would repeat itself for the rest of her life, through her pain, Mimi joined the party, laughing, nurturing others, smiling, wearing a pig nose, and eating her first solid food—chocolate cake.

She started on chemotherapy almost immediately. In ten years, she never went into remission and was never off of chemo except for surgery or radiation. Over the first year, she was in the hospital ten times, five of them for surgery. In December of 1994, she had an unrelated, large brain tumor removed. In the spring of 1995, we all traipsed to L.A. where they took out her liver, removed the last two metastases, and put the liver back in. She had an adrenal gland removed, followed by a very difficult and prolonged recovery. She later had the kidney on the same side removed.

She lost her hair three times, had radiation therapy three times, and four days out of seven, she was sick from chemotherapy. By this year, the constant chemotherapy had taken such a toll on her body that it was starting to wear out. She was experiencing increasing back pain, and in October she developed difficulty expressing herself and mental confusion. Scans showed at least two metastases to her brain and she had surgery to remove one. Radiation and steroids brought back her mental function. By Christmas week, she was in congestive heart failure. She had lung metastases for about a year, and they had finally grown so large that her lung function was compromised. We brought her home on oxygen.

This recital is profoundly depressing, but only serves to emphasize how high above her troubles she rose. She never dwelled on her illness, never felt sorry for herself. She did not just survive her cancer, but she lived a full life.

She touched so many lives in so many ways. This and her children are her legacy. Through her writing and actions, she impacted many lives and set an example of hope and courage. She was selfless. No matter how sick she felt, she was always willing to help and comfort others.

At the cancer center, she always set an example with her positive attitude and smile. She did more than that, however, she would talk to other patients and help them through hard times with the example of her courage, hope, and abounding love. She helped families cope with the death of wives, mothers, fathers, and husbands. She met a young mother blessed with triplets and became her friend, babysitter, and confidant. She became such a part of their lives that that only recently did the children realize that she was not related to them. She advised and guided. She befriended and loved. She was a teacher and cheerleader. She counseled. She saw goodness and potential. She inspired a friend to reconcile with his dying father. She met a young woman outside church, befriended her, helped her improve her English, encouraged her, and inspired her to rise above a menial job and regain the professional state she had trained for. She supported many of you through troubled times.

Most importantly she has taught others to do the same. Everyone she knew has become more loving, generous, and giving from knowing her.

Her other legacy is her children. This was supposed to be a Christmas letter, and I should fill you in on them and the last several years.

Christine is in family practice in Bakersfield. Most of the people working at my office are her patients, and they all love her. She is a very good and caring doctor. She has her own house and is active in her church youth group and choir. She is leading a house-building group to Mexico this spring.

Katie lives in Long Beach with her new husband, Jeff. The wedding was officially scheduled for March, but when Mimi's condition deteriorated, we held an early ceremony on January 24 at the house so she could be there. Katie is a pediatrician and is just starting her practice. Jeff is a photojournalist at the Long Beach Press Telegram. You can see his work at www.jeffgritchen.com. Wedding pictures are at www. jeffkatie.com

David is living in San Diego and still working as a systems engineer for Sun Microsystems. He got his own apartment this year and keeps busy—learning to surf, working, and dating Robin. He has a patent pending and has written two books on computer administration. He is currently taking night classes in business.

Liz graduated from college in occupational therapy and moved back to Bakersfield. She was working for HealthSouth but had an on the job injury and needed neck surgery. She is currently retraining to do marriage and family therapy and is angling for a job at the cancer center when she is done. She just moved into a new house and did a 109-mile charity bike ride last year. More impressive was the 50-mile training runs three times a week.

We are so proud of our children.

═══════════════

Hopefully, Mimi's other legacy will be a scholarship fund. She always did for others, and we hope to continue her work and channel your love and support into something permanent. While plans are not final, the "Mimi Deeths' Memorial Fund" will provide a scholarship for a medical student interested in oncology.

Finally, you all know what a fine writer she was, and we would like to collect her letters and essays. Many of them are in our computers, but we do not have copies of the handwritten ones. If you have saved writings that you would like to share, we would appreciate copies.

May the blessings of God be with you and your families. May the gentleness of spirit, faith in God, and boundless love of Mimi inspire you to share your own love with your family, friends, and others.

Tony Deeths and Family

Appropriately, Mimi's funeral was on Valentine's Day. Almost 700 people came to the Mass, and 60 or more cars followed her to the cemetery. Truly a sign of the respect she deserved.

We thank you all. For the love you have shown us. For the kind words you have expressed. For the meals you have cooked and brought over. For the flowers you have sent. For contributing to her memorial fund. For preparing the final reception in her honor. For the spiritual remembrances you have requested. We thank you for being there.

Introduction

1996

This is Mimi's hope for you in reading this book.

When I was first diagnosed with cancer, my oncologist met with me and my family in my hospital room and outlined his plan of treatment for us. He promised he would do his best to help me in every way medically possible. Then he said there were three other areas, which science was unable to measure, but he felt they were equally as important to my recovery as anything he would provide. These three areas were attitude, support group, and faith.

I have thought about this conversation many times during my recovery, and I feel fortunate to have been blessed in all three areas. First, I was brought up by very dedicated and loving parents who nurtured and encouraged my value as a person. I sought positive-thinking friends as I grew older. My attitude became one of optimism. Second, my childhood was spent among a very close-knit nuclear and extended family that loved and affirmed me as I grew up. That affirmation and bond of affection was so important to me that when my husband and I raised our own children, we worked to develop that type of support among our family and friends. Third, my parents nurtured my faith development until I became mature enough to seek God on my own. That quest is eternal.

I would encourage any readers of this book, at whatever stage in life you are, to take inventory of these three areas of your life. Look carefully at your attitude, your support group, and your faith development. Work on them. Challenge yourself to be the best you can be. When you are working at being a good person, you have a positive attitude about your effort. When you are positive about whom you are, other good people are drawn to you, and when you are surrounded by good people, you begin to understand love. When you grasp the meaning of love, you can begin to comprehend God. The three are intertwined—attitude, support group, and faith.

Develop a sense of humor. Learn to laugh at yourself. Easy for me. I lived with clowns. Mom challenged them. Dad enjoyed them. Work at faith with the same intensity you work at other priorities. Don't just let faith happen, cultivate it.

1996

These are Mimi's thoughts in writing this book.

Today was satisfying and encouraging. I found a group of talented and creative ladies who understand the Spirit and want to write. I'm fired up. I'm inspired!

Tonight I talked to my friend, Kip. Kip is a deep thinker. He takes religion seriously; although it's not any religion I know.

Kip knows my medical situation. He encourages me to take an active part in my medical decisions—to work with and cooperate with the medical professionals. He and I both understand the attitudes of good physicians. They are dedicated, devoted, and caring—and they give up a lot to help others.

Kip knows about visual imagery. He likes to approach disease POSITIVELY. He doesn't like the negative images (i.e. battle, war). You can view your body's immune system and chemotherapy as a battle ground—good cells vs. bad cells, winners and losers, explosions, big fish swallowing little fish, etc.—or you can focus on a positive image. You can seek and find an image of strength, a meaning for life, someone or something bigger than yourself. You can reach beyond the imagery to the IMAGE (God).

He creates, He controls, and He mends. His Spirit lives within me and rises above my fears and encompasses my insecurities. I understand pain and acknowledge suffering because of His Son. I can live because the Spirit of God lives within me, and I can reach beyond myself because God lives outside of me. You (I) don't lose with this arrangement. I never would have thought of such a fancy set-up, but God did.

Now I have to figure out how to put a God that big into a book small enough to sit on a bookshelf, simple enough to be understood, and satisfying enough to be appreciated. What are those three important "D" words we spoke of in the Writer's workshop? Discipline, Determination, Dedication. I would like to add Devotion, and make it four words. These are intense words. At first I viewed them as burdens, hard school master-type words. Discipline is hard, Determination takes a lot of energy, Dedication dictates a mental demand, and Devotion demands a religious dimension. A further consideration of these words, however, reveals to me that they are not burdens but GIFTS. I shall pray for their presence as I spell out my story . . .

CHAPTER 1

Mimi's History

I first met her through my wife. She had a story to share, and little did I realize then, she would become part of my story. I often wonder why she came into our lives. I believe others gift us, and she would share her gifts with us. She was present to us often, and I came to know her. I could see the sickness in her eyes, but I could also see her spirit, her love of life, family, and friends. Her embrace was warm, sincere, and often. She embraced life with that same zeal and determination. She simply wanted each and every day to be a masterpiece, regardless of her circumstances. I learned from her the value of friendship, of reaching out to others, of giving of oneself. She embraced life and everyone around her. I look around my home and see reminders of her. It may be a photograph, a decorative picture, or something as simple as a refrigerator magnetic with the phrase, "Believe in the Magic of Life." She believed, and we who were touched by her presence in our lives have a little better understanding of the magic of life. In the calmness of early morning, as I pray to my God, I think of Mimi and ask the Lord to help me make a masterpiece of this day.

Brad Webb
Friend of Mimi
Husband of Cindy & Father of the triplets—
Riley, Samantha, and Zachary

MY TESTIMONY: MAY 1995

In 1995, Mimi was part of Bible Study Fellowship, BSF.
The last meeting of the year was testimony night.
The members of the group were asked to come prepared
to share a short testimony.
Mimi sat down to think about her past year.
(This is what she wrote.)

Eleven months ago, I was diagnosed with colon cancer. I was operated on, and during that process, the surgeon discovered that the cancer had spread to my liver also. Because there were so many tumors in and on my liver, there was no attempt to do further surgery. I had inoperable liver cancer.

In those days immediately following surgery, I was surrounded by my family of husband and three daughters and a son, all young adults. We were all shocked and stunned. As I emerged from anesthesia and morphine, I sort of chose to isolate myself. It hurt too much to share this burden with the ones I loved. I would have felt alone except in such a situation, morphine is your friend. It takes away pain; it dulls your senses.

Somewhere there in my quietude, the spirit of God replaced the affects of morphine. I quietly accepted His will, I think . . . but I really didn't want his will to be a premature death for me. I had always prayed that I would stay healthy until my children were raised. "Did God misunderstand me?" I wondered. I didn't mean stay healthy just to the minute they were all independent. I meant *at least* that long . . . and then some, like I wanted family dinners at my house with grandchildren someday. I made this clear to God, never more so than on my birthday.

My birthday was three days after surgery, and I woke up feeling sorry for myself. Here I was 45 years old with very little future left . . . it seemed. I was on a stupid IV and couldn't even eat birthday cake! Slight consolation was the fact that my son had flown back to Chicago where I was supposed to be for a family reunion and I knew he would be eating my birthday cake there for me.

My attitude turned around, however, when I received surprise visits from my BSF crew. Batty came and then my discussion leader

Shirley came. I didn't know that they knew . . . but my true sister-in-Christ, Amparo, had told them. Amparo seldom left my side in these days, prayed for me unceasingly, and ministered to my family, which I really appreciated in their time of need. Seeing Amparo and Shirley and Betty flipped my morphine sedated brain to a higher place. They came to me when they, too, must have been afraid, but they shone with the Spirit and their presence alone recalled to me the God I'd learned about in the Minor Prophets, Matthew, and Life and Letters of Paul. He was a personal God, a God of mercy, of Compassion, of Loving kindness. I could approach Him . . . and I did.

That afternoon, my three daughters appeared in my hospital room—3 days after surgery—in celebration mode, laughing and giggling with one another, trying to make me laugh too. I just gave my morphine button a few extra pushes so I wouldn't feel the stitches, and I did laugh with them. They decorated my room, brought party hats, blowers, squeaky balloons, and even birthday cake . . . chocolate (my favorite); I proudly ate as my first solid food . . . after having 15 inches of colon removed. Somehow when you have cancer you learn to put things in perspective—the risk of developing diarrhea seemed worth the chocolate cake. It was. I had no serious digestive problems . . . so I knew God was on my side. I began to interact with Him as a friend in a way I never had before . . .

I asked Him to please let me see my daughters graduate. Ironically, all three of them would graduate that following spring—Elizabeth from high school, Katie from college, and Christine from medical school. (Praise God I am now only weeks from seeing that dream come true).

I had another surprise party in my room that day. My friends from church came and brought me love and laughter and presents. There were not tears, only joy. There was no despair, only hope. They convinced me then and there that life goes on . . . and it does . . .

I received numerous phone calls and encouragement from family and friends out of town . . . and then came the practical reality of dealing with the oncologist. Cancer has a bad reputation, but this doctor battles with it everyday and he believes in his medicine. He also pointed out to me and my whole family assembled that although he would do everything medically possible for me, there were three other things necessary for my cure and here stood our part of the bargain. We would all work together on our attitude, our support group, and most importantly OUR FAITH. The oncologist's visit at the hospital marked the close of my birthday. It was one of my best ever. A time to remember. I knew I was going to make it.

I needed more surgery before chemotherapy began in order to place internal catheters into my blood vessels. All went well with this procedure. I felt in God's hand in this. I started chemotherapy and felt protected in this. I had little discomfort, just slept a lot, drifting off to sleep with quiet spiritual music playing in the background. It was a peaceful time.

That didn't last too long, however; in November, I began to develop vision problems. A trip to my internist and eye doctor revealed trouble. The eye exam showed swollen optic nerves and pressure behind both eyes. An MRI of my head revealed a large brain tumor in the frontal lobes. One week later I went to surgery. I don't remember much about the week preceding surgery. I was numb. The night before surgery, I came to Bible Study Fellowship because that's where I felt secure. I was unaware that my discussion group knew my predicament, but they did. When I asked for prayers, they were understanding, not shocked. The love in their eyes gave me a confidence I've seldom known.

I was tired but reasonably relaxed as the preparations for surgery were begun. The operation was nearly five hours long, and I'm certain God entered my surgical suite. He stood beside my surgeons as they removed the frontal bones of my skull and penetrated my brain, removing a 5 cm tumor that didn't belong where it was. The doctors carefully dissected the tumor from my eyes, my brain, my sinuses, and my pituitary gland. God used the surgeon as his servant—a master surgeon to carry out his Master plan. He is a wise, humble man. I spent 24 hours in intensive care and then 24 hours in a private room watched carefully by my family members in shifts lest I should suffer a seizure. Far from seizure, I was seized by the generosity of God in giving me my children that were home from med school and college to be with me. I had no seizures. I had no pain. I only felt the love. I left the hospital 48 hours later to spend Thanksgiving Day with the family and Katie's roommate Bree who came to share our Thanksgiving. I used no pain killers whatsoever. I didn't need them. Jesus the Comforter was at my side.

Perhaps the hardest part of brain surgery was accommodating to the antiseizure medication I had to be on. One drug made me hyper where I couldn't settle down; the other slowed my brain circuits down so my reflexes were exceedingly slow. I was afraid to leave the familiar environment of my home alone. I couldn't drive my car for three months.

The beauty of this time, however, is that I had to learn to rely on family members and friends to help me. It was a humbling time but a wonderful time of knowing kindness and caring. I came to accept and to understand that this, too, was part of God's plan. Although I've previously been mostly on the giving end of comfort, I was seeing a larger picture here. I was being used as God's tool to bring His Words to life. "For I was hungry and you gave me something to eat, I was thirsty and you gave me something to drink, I was a stranger and you invited me in, I needed clothes and you clothed me, I was sick and you looked after me, I was in prison and you came to visit me.'

"Then the righteous will answer him, 'Lord, when did we see you hungry and feed you, or thirsty and give you something to drink? When did we see you a stranger and invite you in, or needing clothes and clothe you? When did we see you sick or in prison and go to visit you?'

"The King will reply, 'I tell you the truth, whatever you did for one of the least of these brothers of mine, you did for me.' " (Matt 25: 35–40)

In other words, the Scriptures came very alive to me at this time. When one has brain surgery, the brain must do some reorganization and healing afterwards. The electrical nature of the central switch board of out bodies causes your head and nerves to buzz. I was wired! I would lie in bed in the dark of night and feel my brain healing. Sometimes, it would get so loud and so vigorous that my trunk and limbs would buzz. My body felt like a conjunction of fluorescent light bulbs. I couldn't sleep. It was neat, but it could be agitating.

One of the first times this happened to me, I remember feeling scared. I didn't know what was happening. Tony, my husband, was asleep next to me. I didn't want to wake him, but I was afraid I was going to circuit overload and would soon blow a fuse. Suddenly, from the resources of my mind, or the Spirit, or the intervention of a loving Father, I clearly heard the words, "Be still and know that I am God." (Psalm 46:10) Immediately, I felt a gentle warmth course through my veins. I was totally calm, entirely unafraid, and felt cradled in the arms of my Father as I drifted off to sleep.

Another night during this same time period, I was awakened at 2:12 A.M. by a vivid picture in my mind of Jesus walking among the people and curing the sick, casting out demons, raising the dead, and healing the blind man. I recalled my recovery room episodes emerging from anesthesia totally coherent. I recalled the night before surgery when my blind eyes could suddenly see again. I was immediately struck with awe. I couldn't hold it in. I had to wake Tony and tell him of my vision. Crying, I said to him, "I know I'm going to be okay. I am a modern day miracle . . ." Tony said simply, "I know." See what I mean now about being humbled?

I seemed to go through the whole Advent and Christmas season in a state of ecstasy. I was happy writing out my Christmas cards—Tony's letter was cute as usual. I got beautiful notes and prayers back from family and friends. My oldest daughter, Christine, was home from med school and interviewing up and down the whole state of California for residency programs in family practice. On her days off, she did all my Christmas shopping for me—and she wrapped the stuff too. It was a joy for her; it was a delight for me. In addition, I had company every single day. Since I had to be watched constantly for seizures, I had friends come over each day in 3–4 hour shifts . . . until Tony or Liz returned home. It was a great time to pause in the bustle of the pre-Christmas season and visit and reflect. I pulled from resources of friends I never knew I had. Everyone was happy to help me. My house was decorated with poinsettias, like a church lovingly set there by Tony and my friends.

Christmas was wonderful. All four kids were home. Tony's mom and dad and sister joined us for the day. Jesus is the reason for the season. I could see Him everywhere.

Things went well after Christmas. Katie and David were both home for several weeks. Though Chris had to head back to school, the other three kids kept things hopping. The house was alive with young people, and I could shock them with my new hairdo—the basic baldy, post-brain surgery. Kids are great—Wes Fredrick's comment was cool—"All right Mrs. Deeths, way to make a statement!" This was from the mouth of a Berkeley boy. I love these kids; they're so open.

As New Year's rolled around, I began to anticipate a visit from my brother Bill and his wife Nella, whom I'd not seen in nearly three years though we talked on the phone. The only best way to describe these two is family oriented, hard-working, and very, very kind. I greeted them when they arrived from Chicago, made a nice dinner for them on Saturday night, saw Katie and David off to college on Sunday, and after posing for pictures (which I don't remember) I went to bed for a rest. I don't remember going to bed; I don't remember being in bed. I became very ill. The problem seems to have been a combination of chemotherapy, recent brain surgery, anti-seizure medication, antinausea medication, pain killers, dehydration, fever, and electrolyte imbalance.

I was in bad shape, but I didn't know it. I was unaware of the passage of time, mostly because of the constant care given me by Tony, Liz, Bill, Nella (who were staying at our house), and my friends who stopped by. I was too weak to get out of bed by myself so they were helping me walk to the bathroom. When I was too weak to move or unaware of what was happening and had accidents in the bed, they just cleaned up the mess and changed the sheets around me. I was unaware of all this ministering. I was lost somewhere in the recesses of my mind. Nurses came to my home to administer IV's, and though I vaguely recall some of them being there, I was unable to comprehend my situation. Finally, on Thursday of that week, after my brother and his wife left, I was being treated by three friends—Betty, Amparo, and Mary. The Spirit must have spoken to them; they understood the gravity of my illness and called my husband at work and insisted that I be admitted to the hospital. With lightening speed, it seemed this was accomplished. They helped me get ready, Tony came home with a wheelchair, and I was whisked off to Memorial.

I slept on and off for the first five days, hooked up to IV's, packed on ice to get my fever down, and going for diagnostic tests to figure out what was wrong. Nothing was ever conclusive. Then on the morning of the sixth day, my condition turned around. My head was clear; I felt much better. My oncologist cheerfully announced that my white blood cells and potassium levels were up. No one really knew why, but I think I do . . .

About a week after I was released from the hospital, I called my friend, Mary Lue, in St. Louis. I was relaying the events of my latest medical challenge. I mentioned to her how my condition suddenly changed itself on the sixth day . . . There was a long pause on Mary Lue's end of the phone line and then she said, "Oh, God, Mimi, that is the day Janie (her daughter) placed your name at the Wailing Wall in Jerusalem. She carried several names of parishioners, family members, and you from St. Louis on her tour of the Holy Land." Janie is an elementary, religious education teacher now, who used to baby-sit for our four kids. I had no idea she was touring the Holy Land. She had no idea I was as sick as I was at the time.

I received many Mass cards and spiritual enrollments from friends at this time. I felt the power of prayers. It was potent medicine for me.

Soon after this, I had a visit with my neurosurgeon, and frustrated, I told him that my reflexes seemed slow; I wasn't driving yet (nine weeks after surgery), and I just seemed out of it. I thought my brain was not healing well. He patiently assured me it was not my brain but the anti-seizure medication that was creating what he called a *distant personality*. He said I could wean off the medication. This was a most amazing sensation. As I weaned myself over the next week, my distant personality began to merge with my close-up and personal self, and I became one person again and no longer experienced life through my shadow self.

This was another high point for me. Because of my recent hospitalization, I was off chemotherapy still, and now I was off the brain drugs too. I was getting back to becoming the person I used to know. Tony and I escaped for a week to Hawaii together, and I truly became replenished. The past eight months had taken their subtle toll on my nerves. Now they could relax . . .

But not for long—I remember returning home at 3:30 A.M. from the L.A. airport via the late night Bakersfield bus—and glancing at the telephone messages from the week we'd been gone. Blazing out from that list was a friendly message from my oncologist: It made my eyes burn. While I was gone he had scheduled preliminary tests and liver surgery for me at UCLA beginning five days later. (Talk about a fast trip down from a Hawaii high.) I thought I'd throw up. I didn't like this news at 3:30 A.M.

So I went to Mass later that morning and the peace there began to assuage my fears. I got my BSF crew to pray for me on Monday evening, and the following Friday, I found myself in a bed at UCLA Medical Center. The preliminaries for surgery were blessed by a visit from another Bakersfield resident whose husband was on the oncology floor right down the hall from my room. She was very encouraging, offered me some healing tapes, some prayers, and wished me well in surgery the next morning. The next time I saw this wonderful women was back in Bakersfield nine days later, and it was at her husband funeral here in town. Marc, at the age of 40, had died of pancreatic cancer at UCLA while I lie recovering down the hall from him after my liver surgery. At his funeral mass sitting beside my friend, Mary, I had to reflect on life. Why did Marc die so young? Why do I live? These are questions that I keep asking myself. The answer is simply that only God knows the best time for us to die, only in Heaven will his answers be revealed to us. In the meantime, we all must keep answering the question, "Why do I live?" I believe there is only one answer: to give honor and glory to God, Master Creator.

I have to say one more thing about UCLA. It was a good experience. I had never been at a teaching hospital before, but I came to appreciate the internal cooperation, teaching, and feedback of the total staff. They are curious, devoted, and caring. I was assigned a 23-year-old female medical student who came to visit and check my status every morning before 7:00 o'clock staff rounds and every evening before 4:00 o'clock staff rounds. In her, I saw my own daughter, also a 23-year-old female medical student . . . and for the first time, I began to really understand what she did to experience and learn the art of medicine. I could see the student eagerness, the resident approval, and the staff reassurance. I'm proud to have a daughter in medicine.

I marvel still at the way God provides. One of my fears about going to UCLA is that I would be far from my family and friends when I needed them and that Tony would be stressed out trying to juggle work and hospital visits two hours away. No need to worry. Tony was able to take two days off work for the surgery day and my first day in intensive care. He was close by at Tiverton House, a comforting hotel right on the UCLA campus. Katie, our daughter, came from school in San Diego to keep Tony company and oversee my move from intensive care to the step-down unit after Tony returned to work. Katie could only spend a day and a half because of her demanding class schedule, but when she left, I was blessed by the appearance of another angel. My friend, Mary, whose husband was out of town on business that week, drove down and took a room at the Tiverton house and stayed for three days to watch over me and help me out. She provided great comfort, too, to my friend whose husband had the pancreatic cancer. Mary had lunch with Sylvia and her young daughter on the day Marc died. She is the one who drove me and accompanied me to Marc's funeral five days later at home.

Phone calls, family, friends, flowers, and prayers filled the remainder of my days at UCLA. One stunning Sunday, Amparo and I shared the Spirit. She was healing from sinus and nose surgery at home while I was recovering from liver surgery at UCLA. We awoke Sunday morning before 9 A.M., read the same words in *Living Faith*, and simultaneously called one another to share our inspiration. It was a powerful moment on the phone as we shared the reflection.

In addition, we had each read Psalm 91 that morning . . . and we shared part of the Psalm that spoke most clearly to us that day. Amparo felt verses 10–12 because she had been tenderly cared for in convalescence by some special angels just as God had promised:

Then no harm will befall you ,
No disaster will come near your tent.
For he will command his angels concerning you
To guard you in all your ways;
They will lift you up in their hands,
So that you will not strike your foot against the stone.

I had just had successful surgery to remove my last two liver tumors and the surgeon found no further sign of cancer in my body. I was humbled and thankful and the verses spoke to me:

"Because he loves me," says the Lord, "I will rescue him;
I will protect him, for he acknowledges my name.
He will call upon me, and I will answer him;
I will be with him in trouble,
I will deliver him and honor him.
With long life will I satisfy him
And show him my salvation.
Psalm 91:14–16

This section seemed to be my autobiography from especially the past eleven months.

I was awed by this power of the Word. After that day, I shared it with two different Eucharistic ministry teams who had come to the hospital to bring me communion. I was still 'pumped up' by this shared experience of Amparo and me on Monday. That was the day I was scheduled to go home. I thought it would be nice to write a book and share this Spirit with others. I was contemplating this possibility when my new shift nurse walked into the room to introduce himself and begin his patient interview and charting. He was a kind, unhurried man about the same age as me, near as I could tell. He sat down and asked how I was coping with cancer, and I told him the same information I've relayed in these pages. He shared with me that his wife was a cancer survivor and had published a diary of her experiences with breast cancer fifteen years ago. Today, she is a multi-published author and teaches a course in how to write for publication. I have her phone number and her husband's invitation to call her anytime . . . surely this meeting was more than coincidence. It's only another of God's wonderful designs . . .

I believe this testimony is meant to provide the basis for the book I'm writing and eventually, hope to publish. My life is meant to be lived FOR THE GREATER GLORY OF GOD, and I think I've had a *jump start*. I understand more vividly the meaning of the LIVING WORD. I have learned to love God more through my trials. I have felt His touch. I have seen His love reflected through countless others. Surely, cancer can be a physical burden, but when it brings you closer to the HEART OF GOD, it is a blessing.

Amen

(So be it.)

1997

THE WIG STORY

Mimi wrote this story after brain surgery. It speaks volumes to the humor that was used throughout her ten-year battle with cancer to cope with the stress. The wig was brought out for her second brain surgery as well.

In October of 1994 I noticed that my eyes were getting bad. I suspected that age and eye strain were catching up with me and causing distractions in my field of vision. I called my problem "floaters" or "fuzz balls." When I described this to my husband, he said he had them too, sometimes. So I figured this was normal. I knew I needed glasses, in fact, I had known it for a long time, but I was not in any hurry to get them. My life was just simpler without them, but my vision was beginning to concern me.

Finally, I asked my oncologist if he thought that chemotherapy could possibly be causing eye problems. He answered that he didn't think so but consulted with my internist. The two of them decided that I should see an ophthalmologist. I called the office of the doctor recommended to me and was offered an appointment the following week.

"Next week?" I paused on the phone. " That's too soon," I told the receptionist. "That doesn't give me time to clean my house." She seemed puzzled by my response so I explained that my friends from St. Louis were coming to visit. I said I would prefer an appointment three weeks from now after they returned home.

An appointment was scheduled for three weeks into the future, and that was just fine, because I really didn't want to go anyway. I had gone for eye exams once or twice before, and I hated it when those drops went in, and I didn't like the air puff test for glaucoma. Those two things are even more difficult than trying not to blink when you are having your family picture taken. I like my eyes best when I just don't even have to think about them.

I put any thought of the eye exam out of my head and got busy planning a fun itinerary for when my four friends came. We had all met as young mothers eighteen years ago in St. Louis and had shared so much during that time. I was the only one to have moved out of town. They had never been to California before, and I looked forward to showing them the sights. On the day before their arrival, I had my regularly scheduled two-hour intravenous chemotherapy treatment.

Then I figured I would be free of any more trips to the doctor's office for the few days they were here. Generally, I am up and about the day after my treatments, so I was rather disgruntled when I woke up nauseated that day. I took some medication and went back to sleep until it was almost time to leave for the two-hour drive to the Los Angeles airport to pick them up. Although I was still feeling a bit queasy, I was not about to let this small inconvenience interfere with my plans. I decided to skip dinner for fear it would not settle in my stomach. Experience had taught me that nausea, food, and car rides don't mix well. So I clenched my water bottle as if it were my lifeline. Sipping it slowly as I drove along made me feel like I had control of the situation.

My excitement mounted as I approached the airport, found a good parking space, and navigated my way to their arrival gate. I saw them right away as they emerged from the plane. Any fleeting feeling of nausea was dissipated in the hugs and hearty laughter that followed. I loved the warmth of their friendship. For three days we toured the beautiful coastal cities of California, and then I brought them to Bakersfield and proudly showed them my home and reintroduced them to my family whom they had not seen in three years. I was so busy, energized, and excited that I actually forgot about the numerous surgeries and chemotherapy, which had occupied much of my being for the past four months. They commented several times about how healthy and happy I seemed. They were amazed that chemotherapy had not caused any of my hair to fall out. I was happy about that too.

Five days later, and much too quickly, the time came for their scheduled departure. I drove them back to the Los Angeles airport and we hugged each other good-bye. As I drove the two hours home alone, I had that warm-all-over feeling and I reflected on the thoughtfulness of their visit. They had helped me feel whole again and instilled in me the conviction that I was capable of leading a normal life at least for short periods of time. I reflected on the fifteen years we had shared together in St. Louis, and thanked God for those happy times of loving our husbands and raising our children. All of us have busy, growing families, yet these four friends had arranged their schedules and flown together halfway across the country to carry cheer to a friend. That brought tears to my eyes.

The next day I headed off for my overdue eye exam, which brought tears of a different kind to my eyes. Apparently, those "floaters" I had complained about were anchored. The doctor explained that I had swelling of both my optic nerves and pressure behind both eyes. I wished I hadn't come for this exam. Now I started to feel nervous as

I got the distinct impression that not everyone experienced these kinds of floaters like I did.

Later that night I had an MRI scan of my head. My husband is a radiologist so he made arrangements for my study to be done after office hours. I did not understand why it was essential that this be done right away. Tony, however, is a very efficient person, and much to my chagrin sometimes, he is compelled to accomplish things immediately. He and the MRI technician, Vicki, were the only ones at the office besides me. I was sleeping in the MRI machine, as Vicki operated the control panel and my husband waited for the films to be processed.

When I awoke after my hour dozing during head films, I thought it strange that my husband's partner, Norman, had suddenly appeared. The faces of Tony, Vicki, and Norman were intent as they looked at my brain films hanging from the view box. A tear rolled down Tony's nose, and I knew he couldn't speak. I sensed trouble. Norman spoke to me first and said, "There's good news and there's bad news." I feared the bad news was brain cancer. I didn't want to hear it.

The good news was that there was a brain. The bad news was that there was a large tumor in it. The best news was that it appeared to be benign. The worst news was that it had to be removed. So the following day, my husband and I were consulting with a neurosurgeon. The doctor was soft-spoken, kind, and very precise as he performed a complete neurological exam. I trusted him because of his gentle manner and felt pretty sure I 'passed' his exam. I could see how many fingers he was wiggling in my peripheral vision; I could balance on one foot with my eyes closed. I could feel the tuning forks vibrate when pressed to my bones. I thought I could do everything. Maybe there was no brain tumor after all. Oh how I hoped this tumor talk was all a mistake!

Then the doctor asked, "Have you had any changes in personality, say over the past five years?"

"Now," I thought to myself, "that's a loaded question!" In the past three years our family had undertaken a move halfway across the country, my husband had changed jobs, and I had reentered college after a 20-year hiatus. In addition, I was beginning to experience the 'empty nest syndrome' as our two oldest daughters were already away at college, and the younger two teenagers were too quickly moving through high school. I thought these feelings were probably pre-menopausal. In addition, I had also had major back surgery; I only recently had emerged from a year in a back brace. I had gained fifteen pounds mostly from lack of activity, and that made me furious. Five months prior to this day, I had been diagnosed with metastatic colon cancer and had been hospitalized four times for various surgical procedures related to the cancer, and this doctor was asking me if I had had any personality changes?

He waited for my answer. I said, "No, I don't think I have had any *major* personality changes." I certainly didn't want to open up my whole life to this stranger. He was acting like a psychiatrist, and I wondered how much people in his specialty knew about what is inside a patient's head. If I took a lie detector test right now, I wondered if I would fail. Things were happening too fast. I couldn't think straight anymore and wanted to get out of that office.

I was still contemplating whether I should have answered that question about personality more honestly. Apparently, the doctor was discussing surgery with my husband and me. Evidently, I was tuning it out because I suddenly startled when I heard this neurosurgeon say, "There is no acute emergency. You can choose to do the brain surgery anytime within the next two weeks."

"NO EMERGENCY! THE NEXT TWO WEEKS!" Those two sentences didn't go together. This was an emergency! I was hearing **BRAIN SURGERY.**' I don't even like to bang my head, let alone have it cut open and have people moving stuff around inside. I could not even comprehend this latest news.

At this point I think I went numb. The whole thing was more than I cared to understand. Brain surgery . . . bald . . . BAD! I think I got through the next week in shock and only by the Grace of God guiding me. The only emergency I could comprehend in this whole situation was this: How would I cover up my bald head so no one would know? (This is how shallow my thinking had become. Maybe I did need that brain surgery after all!) The next week I scheduled an appointment for myself at Tress Chic Wig Salon. I wouldn't let anybody come with me. I didn't even tell anybody about it. They weren't concerned about my imminent baldness—I was.

I walked into Tress Chic and the owner was very welcoming. She invited me to look around at the variety of wigs on display. I looked around and tried to get enthusiastic about the wigs, but I knew I was going to hate wearing one. "They all look dumb," I thought to myself, and those heads they put the wigs on—well, they look fake. So do the hairstyles."

As my frustration was mounting, a young, red-headed woman walked by me and smiled. I smiled back as she passed by, and I saw her disappear into an adjacent room. When I later looked in that room—oh, my goodness, I couldn't believe my eyes! That young girl with beautiful, long, red hair who had just walked by me in the wig room was sitting in one of the salon chairs, but now she was a woman my age with short stuck-to-her-head gray hair! In real life, she was OLD, but she looked like a teenager in that long, red wig. Things were looking up—if she could look that good in a red wig, why then, so could I. Didn't my hair have a tinge of red? Well, of course, it did—red tint is what I ordered up every six weeks at my hairdresser's shop.

My mistake was going by myself to buy a wig, given my current state of mind. I picked a nice, red one and had it cut and shaped. The salon operator was very kind and kept telling me I looked good. Me—what did I know? I told you my eyes were bad to begin with. I just needed a wig. I thought maybe the wig would make the brain surgery go away.

Confidently, I wore the wig home from the salon. On top of my thick head of hair, the wig took on some extra height. I couldn't fit under the roof of my car without squishing the wig down on my head. What I didn't realize, as I drove along, is that the car roof and my new wig were producing static electricity together, so my new hair was standing upright by the time I arrived at home. It was dinnertime at our house, and my husband and daughter, Liz, were already seated around the table. I sat down proudly with my new, red wig. My husband took one look and rolled his eyes back in his head. My daughter shot a quick glance at her father, and the two of them could not contain their laughter. I was so deflated.

Then Liz said, "Mom, it just doesn't look like you!" My husband agreed that it didn't look like anybody he knew either. For a minute, even I wondered who I was. I got up from the table to look in the bathroom mirror. Oh, it did look like a fright wig! I didn't know whether to laugh or cry, but I figured I had too much trauma ahead of me to start my crying now so I decided to laugh with them. Then the joking started one of the goofiest, yet loving evenings that I can recall. Tony and Elizabeth decided that since I was going to change my appearance so drastically, they would ask the neurosurgeon to change my personality too.

They placed the neurosurgeon in the role of the mad scientist, and imagined they would ask him to create a new woman. Since I am not known for my aptitude in cleaning house, my husband was going to have the surgeon deliver subliminal messages to my brain during surgery and create a wife who loved to clean. Our oldest daughter, Christine, had been granted a leave of absence from her medical school, and she arrived home this evening and joined in the family scenario. We spoke to our other two college children by phone that night and they, along with Christine and Elizabeth, contributed their ideas toward creating the ideal woman. The kids were going to program a mom who loved to cook every night and let them have her car because she was anchored in the kitchen. She would make regular trips to the post office to send letters and care packages to her hard working, starving son and daughters away at school. The new woman was going to be sexy and wear revealing outfits to go along with that new, red wig. As the evening drifted into a fairy tale, there was a happy ending. They all loved me just the way I was now, and they wanted that same wife and mother back after brain surgery. Our family sometimes has a rather bizarre sense of humor, but what we had all been doing was to try to survive this difficult week while we waited and wondered and worried.

My friends from church also helped me survive that week. There were things too difficult for me to share with my family, but I could talk them over with my close friends. Expressing my fears to my family was one thing I would not do because I felt they already had enough to deal with. I was afraid I might become a burden to them, and I did not want to vocalize my concern that I might become helpless and dependent. I wanted so badly to remain a vital part of the world I knew. Three days before surgery, five of these faith-filled friends joined me at church to pray for God's guidance for my physicians, for my healing, and for my family's strength. At lunch later that day, I had told them all about the little 'reprogramming' joke being carried on at home. One of my friends, Carolyn, brought along a movie camera, and they decided to interview me on camera at the restaurant. "In this way," they said, "you will be able to look back on these movies and remember how you used to be prior to your reprogramming."

My friends were carrying on the reprogramming plan that my family had begun at home. We were all getting carried away with it as we laughed and created funny visions in our heads. Then I remembered that it was my head we were all referring to, and the reality crept in. I had been told by the surgeon that I might suffer some temporary memory loss as a result of the surgery. My fear was that I might not recognize my family upon awakening from the anesthesia. That thought left me feeling totally out of control and very frightened. My friends understood and listened lovingly as I verbalized my insecurities. There is not too much that even good friends can do in a situation like this. Later that evening, however, my friend, Carolyn, gave me all that she could. She came to my house and dropped off the silly movie she had made for me that afternoon. I watched it and laughed until the end when her sincerity welled in my heart. Attached to the end of the film was a video scene that Carolyn and her husband had spliced in for me. The scene was Carolyn, with her strong angelic voice, singing one of my favorite songs from the church choir, beginning and ending with the words, "You are, Oh God, my inheritance, You are all I need." Those words were the gift I needed most.

On the day before surgery, I could not settle down. I was sad at home because I was afraid that this familiar family scene, which I loved so much, would be taken away from me. Since I felt that getting away might ease my nervousness, I went to my Monday night Bible Study because I always felt secure there. When I entered my small discussion group, I was unaware that most of the ladies already knew I was having brain surgery the next morning. I found out later that one of my friends had informed the group before I arrived. When I asked for their prayers, they were sympathetic, not shocked. The love in their eyes gave me a confidence I have seldom known. I told them that I would be rising the next morning for a 5:30 A.M. hospital check-in and was afraid to leave my house, for fear I might not recognize it after my surgery. One of my discussion group members responded, "Then I will be down on my knees praying for you at 5:00 tomorrow morning so you will be able to leave and return to the same house you have always known. I will pray all morning for the success of your surgery and for your complete recovery." The rest of the group promised me their prayerful support, and I left Bible Study that night enveloped in love after receiving a group hug and prayer from the leadership staff. Another very amazing thing happened that night. My friend, Amparo, who also attends Bible Study felt compelled to follow me home that night. You have to know Amparo and the way she drives. She has one speed usually, and that is fast. She started quickly out of the parking lot, as I did my usual dawdling. She was far ahead on the road, when I suddenly realized that I was overtaking her. She continued to poke along and filed into the traffic lane behind me. I thought she was just goofing around, but she told me the next day that the Holy Spirit warned her to follow me because I may not be safe. As we came to my subdivision entrance, she pulled along side me and waved good-bye.

I waved back in a wild, mocking sort of way and laughed at her for her silly idea to follow me home. Then I turned quickly onto my street. My head began spinning; my eyes went fuzzy. By the time I eased my car to a safe curb area, my eyes were blind. Alone in the dark I understood now that the surgery was necessary and imminently so.

My vision returned quickly as I pleaded for my sight back and turned my head heavenward. I took this as a sign of God's awareness and protection of me. I had prayed for signs before. He always answered my need.

The next morning, I was able to kiss my daughters, Christine and Elizabeth, good-bye and leave my home confidently with Tony at 5:15 A.M. I had an aura of peace and acceptance. I wanted to get this job finished. Although I was tired from interrupted sleep, I felt reasonably relaxed as the preparations for surgery began. After I undressed, put on a hospital gown, and climbed into bed, the 'barber' came in and shaved my head smooth with one of those buzz-cut clippers. In about one minute, I went from a thick head of hair to totally shorn. Now I understood how those wooly sheep must feel after shearing. I started to shiver—my head was cold, and I was scared. The anesthesiologist began an intravenous drip and kindly added some sedation to it. That is all I remember until I woke up in the intensive care unit about six hours later. Around my bed were assembled three doctors, a nurse, my husband, and my daughters, Christine and Elizabeth. I could see them. I recognized my family and could feel their concern. One of the doctors asked, "Do you know us?" With three pairs of brown eyes, surgical masks and caps, those doctors all looked the same to me. I said, "No!" because I didn't want to concentrate that much. All I wanted to do was sleep.

After I had rested a while, the neurosurgeon came in again. His first words stated "the tumor was benign; the surgery went very well." For this I was very thankful. The next words I comprehended were, "Now that the blood supply to the vessels in your scalp has been altered, you cannot wear anything binding on your head. No wigs."

My husband had that problem solved quickly. He found a non-binding wig for me. It came in seven fluorescent colors, in alternating stripes, the kind the circus clowns wear. He brought it up to the intensive care unit. They needed some laughter up there, and it brought a smile to the faces of the nurses and other visitors. Tony tried it on to show me how nice it looked. Elizabeth, my daughter, came up to visit after school and put the clown wig on and sat there with a big smile on her face. We made quite a pair—the clown kid and mummy-head mom. The room did not seem serious like I imagined the Intensive Care Unit would be, but I felt nothing but intensive care with a light and loving touch. The clown wig became a symbol of our attitude of family togetherness. The rainbow wig was the sign for bright things to come after the storms of the past few months. It helped the healing begin . . .

Mid-1997

PSALM SECURITY

*Mimi wrote this after her liver surgery at UCLA;
it speaks perfectly to how she turned to God throughout
her entire illness to help her get through the tough times.*

Three years ago I was lying in a hospital bed waiting for the surgeon to come in and tell me the worst was over; the tumor had been removed from my colon, and all I had to do now was recover and go home. Instead, as he stood beside my bed, I heard the word "Cancer" emerge from his lips.

I was drowsy enough from the post-anesthesia effects and intravenous morphine that I believed I just heard the words wrong. I asked groggily for reassurance, "Cancer? Well, you got the whole tumor out, didn't you?"

"Yes, the entire colon mass has been removed," he answered.

I felt a sense of relief as I let my weary body sink back into the bed and muttered a half-hearted "thank you" as I gave the morphine dose button another push. I waited for the surgeon, the burden bearer, to leave the room.

He remained, and the next words I registered were, "The cancer has reached your liver."

Now I really felt like I wanted him to get out of the room, but he didn't look like he was moving toward the door. He seemed to get taller, and I felt I was getting smaller. I wished I could disappear or run away. Hoping to find assistance in my escape plan, I looked to the faces of my husband and my teenage kids who stood at the foot of the bed. They looked too wounded to help me run. I realized at that moment that they probably had already heard the news that was just now sinking into my conscious mind. Their grave faces reinforced the severity of the surgeon's words.

I hated to see them look like that. In our family we like to have fun. We tease each other and laugh a lot. Where were the smiles? Where was the laughter? I tried desperately to bring those cheerful faces back, so this time I looked to the surgeon to help me. I looked up at him with eyes of hope and asked,

"Well did you take my liver out then?

No, you need your liver," was his simple answer.

"Well, did you at least take the bad parts out?" I asked desperately.

His words were calm and precise. "There was too much of it, too much cancer in and on the surface of your liver. Removing them was not feasible."

I looked into his sad eyes and just as quickly looked away. I closed my eyes, hoping this whole scene would be gone when I opened them again.

I don't know how long I was asleep, but when I woke up I knew that this was more than just a bad dream. Whirling inside my head were the words of Psalm 23. These are words I usually heard at funerals as the priest says softly such phrases as "near restful waters . . . He'll give me repose . . . and though I walk through the valley of darkness, no evil should I fear." It seemed strange that funeral words could give me such a sense of peace when I did not want to die.

"Why," I wondered "did these words come to me in my sleep?" I tried to make my mind remember the rest of the words of that Psalm. I recalled that in my student years, teachers had said that the Bible spoke to you. Supposedly, some people are able to simply flip through the Bible, stop on any page, and discover a message specific to them in their current need. I had tried this a few times in the past, and although those words may have been trying to reveal something important to me, they sure didn't make any sense at the time. I had long since stopped the practice of expecting the Bible to produce some sudden inspiration.

Today these Bible words were coming to me in my sleep, and I became very aware that while I slept, the Spirit within me was alive and alert. The Spirit was helping me to remember the rest of the Psalm and now phrases were swiftly sailing into my head. "The Lord is my Shepherd." Yes, indeed that was the opening line. "I shall not want. " I decided then to surrender to the will of God. "Near restful waters He leads me to revive my weakened spirit." Well, isn't that what the steady fluid drip in the intravenous line was doing right now! Then I remembered the words, "Only goodness and kindness will follow me all the days of my life." That was the phrase I needed now. The Bible truly was speaking to me—ALL THE DAYS OF MY LIFE is what it was saying. I knew that meant I was going to live!

Today, I am grateful for the dedicated team of physicians, nurses, family, and friends who helped me through those early months of chemotherapy and further surgeries. My oncologists conferred with one another, with my family, and with me. We agreed to try a combination of treatments due to the extent of my disease. I had more tests and more surgeries. Arterial angiograms were done to study the arrangement of the blood vessels in my body. Another surgery was performed to place a central venous catheter into the major vessel branching from my aorta. A second catheter was placed directly into my liver. Both these catheters would direct the flow of chemotherapy that I would be receiving. One would provide systemic chemotherapy that would circulate through my entire system; the other would carry potent cancer killing drugs directly to my liver. This did not sound like fun, but what other choice did I have? These options brought me hope.

The results of these early months of chemotherapy were, as the doctors called it, "dramatic." Repeated MRI scans showed that the sizes of four tumors in my liver were decreasing. If they could shrink, I had hopes that they could disappear all together. I prayed that the tumors would die so I could live.

Within eight months of my original diagnosis, I lay in a bed on the oncology floor of the UCLA Medical Center. I was scheduled for liver surgery the next morning. I don't remember being very scared. All the pre-op tests had shown that there were only two shrunken masses left in my liver, and the UCLA team was prepared to remove them with a relatively new technique called cryosurgery. This method of freezing the tumor was fairly new. I didn't ask how new, but I heard people tag the word "experimental" to it. Being a "guinea pig" is a scary thought, but I also was fully aware that most scientific advances in medicine occurred through the use of just such willing participants. It was scary, but there was also an element of excitement surrounding the procedure . . . and a whole lot of trust placed in the skill of the surgeon.

I went to surgery surrounded by doctors, nurses, technicians, anesthesiologists, and a team of medical students eager to witness this new technique. I understood then why the Lifetime Channel on TV calls it the operating "theatre." I was center stage and trying hard to control my stage fright so I wouldn't vomit. I quickly glanced around the room, saw no escape, and wished I wasn't the one lying here. Then the anesthesia flowed into my vessels, and I was unaware of anything.

Six hours later, I woke to find myself in one of the intensive care units at UCLA. Talk about a frightening place! You can lay there and listen but not hear anything of human voice. The nurses move around quietly while machine sounds and beeping monitors replace the human sound of voices. I looked around to both sides of my bed and saw two frail aged people who looked like corpses. I hoped I didn't look like that.

As I glanced around this foreign environment searching for a familiar face, I must have succumbed again to the sedated sleepiness following surgery. Then I felt a slight pressure on my toe and looked to the foot of my bed. I saw my surgeon. He had a smile on his face. I'd never seen him smile before. Then he said in a very kindly voice, "I could not have asked for the surgery to have gone any better. Thank you, Mrs. Deeths, you just made my day!"

"I think it goes the other way around." I groggily said, "It's YOU that made my day. Thank you." I would have talked more, but I just wanted to relish his words, and I drifted back off to sleep clinging to this encouraging news.

Recovery was painful as it usually is after surgery, and while I recovered on the oncology floor, I suffered a serious setback to my security. Though my physical condition continued to improve, one of the other patients whom I had come to know on the oncology floor lapsed into a coma and died of his cancer. I became acutely aware of the fragility of human life and became fearful for my own survival. I was treated with kindness and reassurance by every person whom I encountered. Family laughter, encouragement from those back home, the kind assistance of a friend, and staff reassurance helped me gain back a sense of perspective during the week I was hospitalized.

On the day before I was scheduled to leave the hospital, I was awaken for the mandatory vital signs, which the nurses like to do at 6 A.M. I couldn't get back to sleep and was trying to mentally prepare myself for discharge from the hospital. I was anxious to get home and begin my life again though I still had nagging fears about reoccurrence of my cancer. The day was Sunday, and I felt bad that I would not get to Church this day. Out of a sense of guilt, most likely, I reached for my daily devotional packed into the little suitcase beside my bed. I began reading the Scripture passage for the day, Psalm 91. Never again will I doubt that the Bible indeed speaks to the needs of each one of us. In my state of fear and doubt, God Himself addressed my need and through tears of gratitude I read the final verses of this Psalm in which He says,

> "Because he loves me," says the Lord, "I will rescue him;
> I will protect him, for he acknowledges my name.
> He will call upon me, and I will answer him;
> I will be with him in trouble,
> I will deliver him and honor him.

With long life will I satisfy him
And show him my salvation.

Once again the Bible spoke to me and helped bounce me back more fully and more completely into the life He has planned for me.

1997

ADRENAL TUMOR

This story was written in 1996. It shows the frustration and upset of a setback. It shows the decisions of who to tell and when. It speaks of the support and encouragement of family members, and also the hope and confidence in your doctors that you must hold onto.

Because of rising CEA levels for about six months, Dr. Patel and I decided to repeat CT and MRI scans within the next month instead of waiting for the usual six month schedule. My last scans in January had been negative, and I was scheduled to repeat them on April 29 and 30. I did not think too much about them. I have become very used to them. I just sleep inside the machine, no big deal. I had no inkling that there was any questionable area on the scans; nevertheless, I am nervous each time as I await the official dictated report.

Norman was out of town until Wednesday, so I knew the scans would not be read until then. However, Satya took a look at them on Wednesday and questioned an area on the left adrenal gland that appeared to be abnormal. Norman returned to town on Wednesday, but he did not get time to read the new scans and compare them to all my past films. Norman is very intense and prefers to study this type of complicated comparison case when he is alone and uninterrupted. In this busy practice that did not happen until after office hours on Friday.

I will not forget sitting exhaustedly (it had been too many days of anxiety) in the den as Tony answered the phone out on the patio. Through the open screen door I could hear bits and pieces of his conversation. I knew it did not sound hopeful. After Tony hung up the phone, he walked quietly into the den and sat down. He said the conclusion was that there was definitely a mass in the left adrenal, and in reviewing past films, it had been there since shortly after the original cancer diagnosis in June of 1994. Furthermore, it had been growing.

I started to cry. There was such a well of emotion. I felt that I had been cheated. Why hadn't they found it sooner? This cancer had been allowed to grow unnoticed for over a year and a half. I trusted these doctors—why hadn't they found it sooner? Anger was beginning to take over. The radiologists missed it in October of 1994, and again in December. The surgeon didn't look there in March of 1995.

It was missed again on repeat scans that summer of 1995. The rising CEA from January 1996 to April of that same year should have been a tip-off. Why didn't anybody figure it out sooner???? I was feeling hopeless. I remember taking a deep breath, laying my head back, and saying to Tony—this cancer is a hard disease to fight. It isn't fair. He agreed and then sat there silently. One thing I have learned is that each person in my family has to deal with my condition differently. Tony, I think, needs to contemplate . . . and from there arises courage to deal with each situation.

After a time sitting in my chair, I got to thinking that I am a pain. It was not fair that everyone had to suffer with me. I needed reassurance that I was still loved, and I asked Tony an unfair question. After 26 years of marriage, I said, "Do you ever wish that you did not marry me?"

His answer was clear and uncompromising. "No, never." I got up from my chair. I needed to be held and hugged to feel secure.

Katie was not yet home from work, and Christine was due to stop in after her grueling day at the hospital. I knew I had to get control of my emotions before they came home. I was still sitting in the same chair. I just did not have the energy to move. I felt drained. One of the hardest parts of this disease is telling family members.

Katie came in first and had exciting things to report about her day. Katie usually does have some part of her day to share. She's the type of kid who wears her heart on her sleeve. She's a feeler and wants others to know about the little things in today that make it different from another day. She brings energy into a room when she enters. The awareness that she was having an ordinary enthusiastic day while I was recovering from devastating news . . . and that we could both be sitting in the same room, made me realize that my crisis could not bring everybody down. I waited until she finished her daily discourse, and then I quietly asked her to come over and sit on my lap. I still couldn't move from the chair, but I wanted her close to me. I like to feel her energy.

I told Katie that the doctors had found another tumor. Sensible kid that she is, she asked "Where?" When I told her it was on the adrenal, like behind my stomach, she just pointed her index finger like a laser gun at the area and shouted, "Get out of there!" I laughed, and the laughter broke the ice crystals that were hanging on my heart. Then Katie took her hand and made the sign of the cross on my forehead and said, "I'm sorry about it. I am blessing you." I knew then she was o.k. with this. I was becoming more comfortable too.

Christine dropped in for a visit shortly after that, and we told her. Young doctor that she is, she wanted to know all the details and what we were going to do about it. Her father had to answer those questions. I was still in the state of shock. By the next morning Christine had consulted with every available surgeon on the staff at her teaching hospital and had formed all her recommendations for us. I realize more and more how this oldest child of ours has what it takes to be a good physician.

Tony and I made the decision not to tell our two youngest children right away. David was still in school, and there was no need to get him disturbed. Liz had just finished finals and was looking forward to going out with her inter varsity group for two weeks working with the Urban Tacoma Project. We did not want to dampen her spirit for this worthwhile endeavor. I never want to tell my mother because she worries so much and feels totally helpless because she lives 2,000 miles away. Tony's mom and dad are both in their eighties with their own daily difficulties so we elected not to trouble them until we ourselves had come to a decision.

Coming to a wise decision on medical problems such as mine takes time. It had already been five days since I had these scans that revealed the tumor, and it had seemed like an eternity to me. I wanted action immediately, but it was the weekend. So I had to wait to consult with my doctors at least until Monday. This weekend was a hard one for me. I was still frustrated and angry. I wished that I was a long-distance runner. It was 100 degrees outside, but I was ready to take to the bike trail and run those 15 miles from one end of the city to the other in the heat until I was so exhausted that I just dropped and had no energy left over with which to be frustrated and anxious or angry. I felt like a restrained tiger, and all I wanted to do was pounce . . . but I lacked the energy and the initiative.

I was sure that my doctors would react to the printed report of my tumor with as much immediacy as I felt it required. They did not contact me on Monday. They did not contact me on Tuesday. By Wednesday I was hounding my husband—had that X-ray report gone out? He called my oncologist and my internist to see if it had been received. Neither of them had seen the report yet. Oh, I was fired up again—what is wrong with the communication system in this town. Who screwed up?? The typist, the delivery person, the physician's office receptionist? Were the doctors too busy to care??? I had just finished a two-hour chemotherapy treatment. My doctor had not been in the office so I couldn't talk to him. I felt sick. I was depressed. I slept out on the patio lounge chairs and felt the sun and listened to the birds. They were my only friends. I prayed for comfort, but it did not come easily.

One ray of hope occurred during this time. Tony spoke with his brother, an urologist who pointed out that frequently adrenal tumors are benign and do not cause any major problems. They can remain in the body, or if the decision is to remove them, it is a relatively uncomplicated surgery. I trust Jeff's judgment and began to think of this tumor as benign. That made my life easier. Just about the time I was entering complacency, I got a phone call from both my oncologist and internist. They had conferred with one another and felt that there was a reasonable possibility that this tumor was benign. They hoped to spare me from another surgery if this proved to be true. They suggested I have a biopsy of the adrenal gland.

Coward that I am, the thought of a long needle going into the core of my abdomen was terrifying. The good part about this is that the premier radiologist for this particular procedure was out of town for the next four days so I knew I would be spared at least until then. I tried to get this whole tumor problem out of my head. I was progressing as usual on my normal course of chemotherapy and was experiencing some side effects from that. That alone was plenty to deal with and I was able to ignore the thoughts of the tumor.

Tuesday, May 14, dawned and I knew I had to do that biopsy. I called the doctor to schedule it and got his voice mail. When he did not return his voice mail page, I drove over to the hospital and encountered him myself. He was welcoming and polite as usual. I was actually feeling good and the side effects of the previous week's chemotherapy had subsided. I told him I needed that biopsy today. He explained the procedure and said he could schedule it for later that afternoon. I asked him if he used anesthesia for it. When he said no, I asked him if he would prescribe valium to relieve my anxiety. He consented to that so long as I had a designated driver accompany me for this outpatient procedure.

When the doctor showed me my CT scans on the view box and indicated the route through which he would have to pass the needle through my back, I could see the small margin of error. He would be working in about an eighth of an inch clear radius. I had visions of myself jumping off the table, jerking away with the first pierce of the needle, and making blood go all over the place as he punctured a lung or a kidney or something else because I wiggled. That's where the valium helped. It mellowed me out so I was still aware of the procedure being done, but I was too relaxed to react.

The biopsy tissue was removed quickly and sent immediately to the lab for a preliminary reading. Initial readings looked like normal adrenal tissue, so I confidently got up and dressed and left the office to go sleep off my valium at home. Things were looking up.

The next day (Wednesday), I went for week four of chemotherapy as usual. I told the nurses that it appeared that the tumor was benign, and we could just ignore it. In the meantime, I told them, I would add a fifth week to my usual four-week chemotherapy schedule because I was not having much difficulty with side effects. Furthermore, Dr. Patel and I had agreed previously that five or even six weeks was probably desirable, in that it might tend to lower my CEA level. We might be able to kill off another generation of cancer cells . . . wherever they were hiding in my body.

Basically, I began to relax about this tumor. I felt it must be benign, and I resigned myself to additional weeks of chemotherapy to try to get the CEA level down. Life was going on as normal. Tony left the next day (Thursday) for a four-day radiology meeting in Los Angeles. I was sort of worn out from the latest chemo treatment, and it was easy to just rest and relax, no worries about dinner preparation, schedules, etc.

On Friday morning Tony's partner, Don, who had performed the biopsy, called to say that some of the cells in the frozen sections were "suspicious." So much for complacency with this tumor. This meant war! I told him I was not too surprised. It actually might be good. Perhaps we had located the cause of the rising CEA levels. I have become used to waiting things out with this disease. You must learn to be patient. So on the outside I was practicing my patience; on the inside, I was in turmoil.

Tony arrived home late on Sunday after visiting his parents in Los Angeles. I was not feeling well when he arrived home, so we did not discuss the pathology results. The next morning I was still not feeling well so I did not get up with him when he went off to work. That evening, he got home after I had already left for my Bible Study, and it was after 10:00 P.M. when we had our first chance to talk in the past five days.

I asked if he had inquired about my pathology at work that day and he said yes; he had the final report. I said, "Is it metastatic? He said yes; it looked like it was. I was not surprised, and the news actually set me at ease. Bible Study that night had been filled with beautiful testimonials, and I was feeling very much at Peace with my whole life situation. Peace I leave with you. My own Peace I give to you, not the peace that the world gives. This is my gift to you (John 14:27). I felt that it was His gift to me. I had another cancer tumor. It was unsettling but that PEACE He gave to me. It could conquer all. This is what I would cling to during the next weeks of decision making.

I began to prepare myself mentally for the likelihood of surgery. I hated the thought of stronger and longer chemotherapy or new experimental treatments. Surgery was actually sounding like the most desirable option. The question was, do I have it here in town or go back down to UCLA? If it had been simple surgery for a benign tumor, I would have had it here in town for the convenience of myself and my family. We were dealing with a larger entity here. CANCER, by name, needs many smart heads together for problem solving. I was coming to the conclusion that UCLA would be the best choice. In the meantime, I heard from my oncologist who had already scheduled appointments for me with a medical and a surgical oncologist at UCLA.

I continued on chemotherapy weeks five and six and was pleasantly surprised that the side effects were not nearly as severe as I had anticipated. Fatigue and peripheral nerve involvement were the main problems. It was hard to tell how much of this was actually due to chemotherapy and how much was in response to the emotional roller coaster of the last few weeks. I had an appointment with my internist that week, and she was very reassuring. She said my adrenal hormone levels were within normal range. My blood pressure was elevated slightly more than normal, but I didn't think that was significant. I know it was high because of the stress and indecision, anger, frustration, and this period of testing my patience. She liked the idea of surgery. She said I was healthy, tended to recover quickly, and I didn't need that adrenal gland anyway because I had another one on the other side. Personally, I thought she was being a little cavalier with my organs, but I knew that she was being honest. She said it would be interesting to see if the removal of this gland would bring down my CEA. I couldn't wait to see. Surgery was looking like the best option.

A week later was Memorial Day holiday, and we eagerly looked forward to our two youngest children coming home from college. Liz was arriving home after her first year and a two-week experience with the Tacoma Urban Project. I looked forward to seeing her. There was so much I wanted to hear about, but I also knew that her coming meant that I would have to tell her that I had another cancer metastases. I hate to share this, but I have to. It's the only way I can survive it. She was home a while and settled in before I told her. She looked at me with sympathy, yet with the trusting eyes of a child who knew things would turn out all right. That gave me confidence. Liz is a realist. She puts one foot in front of the other everyday and walks through life with inner calm and minimal frustration about those things in life we cannot change. She has taught me a lot. I'm trying to be more like her.

I told David later that same evening. He was sad to hear, but he reacts much like his father and wanted to know what we were going to do about it. My men like to see solutions to life's problems. I told him I didn't know yet, but that I felt sure that things would turn out just fine. He seems secure when I am secure. He was able to go back for his final two weeks of school, finals, apartment hunting for summer school, and clearing out his current apartment. He handled the stress. He's had lots of practice. He'll handle the next step when it comes along.

The following Monday (June 3), I had an appointment with my oncologist who wanted to see me before I went to UCLA. He was encouraged that this appeared to be an isolated tumor, and he was hopeful that it could be successfully removed by surgery. He also felt secure that my two years of chemotherapy had kept this tumor site from growing out of control. I was feeling good even about chemotherapy. I was just feeling pretty positive about life in general . . . until he ordered a bone scan. I thought he had suspicions that there may be bone metastases. That's a scary thought. I could feel my bones hurt! The bone scan was scheduled the following day, and thank God, was negative.

One week after I finished my sixth week of chemotherapy (Friday), I had my consult at UCLA. My daughter Christine took the day off and accompanied me. It's a good thing she did because I was not feeling well that morning, and I slept most of the two-hour ride down. By the time I arrived at UCLA, I was feeling quite well and looked forward to seeing the surgeon. He was very sympathetic when I told him I was back with another tumor. I told him it was in the adrenal gland (not my liver)! He said he would help if he could and ushered me into the office to review my scans and path report. At the end of his exam, he prescribed a PET scan and said he would make his decision on surgery after he looked at the results of those tests. It would be Monday morning before I would get the results. More waiting! What he explained and what increased my anxiety is that he wanted to check for any additional sites of metastases in my organs. If he found multiple metastases, then it would not make any sense to operate on just one site. It wouldn't help me. I was beginning to feel a bit desperate. With all these scans, something bad would surely show up, but God watches over me, and this scan showed nothing. He called my home first thing Monday morning and said he would do the surgery. What a relief, and I knew him and I had confidence in him.

Surgery was scheduled for the following Friday—twelve days away. I had an answer now. I had something to aim toward. It was very reassuring. Mentally, I began to prepare myself, to exercise, to rest, to eat wisely, so I'd be in the best possible condition. My prayer chains were mobilized and friends joined me at Mass to pray during the days preceding surgery. That gave me great comfort. I have the secure feeling that I will be fine. I was able to call my mother and tell her. I felt so confident that this was the answer to all our prayers.

Sept. 2002

LOVE AND APPRECIATION

This was written after Mimi's kidney surgery. She meant to send it out to everyone who helped her. She didn't get them all sent out, so if you are reading this for the first time. Thank you for all you did.

September 28, 2002

I may have lost a kidney, but everywhere I turned I found LOVE, which more than compensated for any loss. I have nothing but thankfulness as I look back on the past five weeks since surgery. I have begun several times to write thank-you notes, but I was truly overwhelmed by the number of friends to whom I would want to write. During the period of recuperation at the hospital and at home, I must say I just allowed myself to lay back and bask in the loving attentiveness of so many.

For those of you interested in the story, read on. For those who already know it or who have heard enough of my stories, you can stop here. Please know how much you are loved and appreciated.

Anyway, for those who don't know the details, my left kidney and surrounding area have been plagued with problems for the past three years. I've had laser surgery, chemotherapy, stint placement in the ureter for proper drainage, and radiation to the area around the kidney. Each procedure worked for a while. However, in the past nine months, scans had revealed that there was a growing tumor in the middle of that kidney that was not responding effectively to chemotherapy. I am blessed that I was born with two kidneys, and only one of them was faulty. I found a great surgeon at UCLA who felt that he could safely remove my cancerous kidney . . . and that's just what he did on August 21.

The surgery took just a little over three hours, and I awoke to a most beautiful sight. Around my bed were seven of my favorite faces: Tony, Christine, Katie, David, Liz, Katie's boyfriend, Jeff, and David's girlfriend, Robin. They had all taken the day off work, spent a night or two in a hotel right there on the UCLA campus, laughed together, and helped Love me back to good health. They were in and out of my room each day. Life doesn't get much better than this. There were even a couple of anonymous people in the recovery and hospital room in the first several hours after surgery. I was given two transfusions immediately after surgery . . . so someone who doesn't even know me cared enough about patients to donate blood. I am ever grateful to them. Initial blood tests show that the blood I received was probably better than my own that I had lost. I don't find that surprising.

I was well taken care of in the hospital. Flowers, balloons, cookies, candy, and company arrived daily. As food for the soul, someone from the local Los Angeles area Catholic Church Hospital ministry brought me Communion and prayed with me each day. Tony and the kids enjoyed escaping together to some of the finest restaurants in Los Angeles. Katie is a pediatric resident right there at UCLA Medical Center so she knows the good places in the area that fit into her father's budget but not hers. I wish I had felt better so I could have gone with them! I was, however, very content to just have that surgery over with and be on the road to recovery. I had visits from Tony's cousin, Joyce, who drove down from her home in Glendale. My brother Bud and his wife, Lynn, drove over from Riverside. "Mother" Gail from San Diego was planning to come visit on Monday (my fifth day in the hospital), but I got promoted before that and was sent home four days after surgery! I still marvel at the wonders of modern medicine, and thank God for the wonderful ability of our bodies to heal.

My surgery had been on a Wednesday that week. By Sunday night, I was home sleeping in my own bed. Tony, Christine, and Liz were all home to help. On Monday, I was overwhelmed with the caring and kindness of my friends. I had phone calls and flowers and deliveries of warm dinners that week. Friends came by and brought me lattes, blenders, and mocha freezes to energize me. Another friend brought me a prayer blanket, which had been made by some of the church ladies and blessed by the priest. It was good to cuddle under it when the caffeine from the mochas wore off. My neighbor who had just returned from Italy brought me some beautiful glass beads from Verona. The beads made me realize that I would be up and around soon and dressed in something besides pajamas.

It didn't take long for that wish to come true. Two weeks after surgery, my first outing was to Church. Just before I had gone to the hospital, our Monsignor had administered the Sacrament of Anointing as my friends offered their prayers for me. Now I was back at Mass and realized that the blessings, successful surgery, and healing that we had all prayed for, had indeed occurred. Faith, hope, and love had indeed been showered upon me. For this I am ever grateful.

Following those first weeks, I worked to wean off the pain medication and build up my strength. I've been back to see the surgeon who seemed genuinely pleased with my progress. I have seen my oncologist here in Bakersfield, and he is happy that we can probably switch to a new type of chemotherapy that will be less toxic to my healthy cells. He's giving me a rest and recuperation time off for good behavior right now, but as always, he is upbeat and encouraging about continuing treatment. I was recently at a dinner and celebration at the Cancer Center here in Bakersfield for the dedication of an interfaith chapel within the building where I go for treatment. My oncologist welcomed the crowd gathered and spoke on what he has learned from his patients. He spoke about the role of faith. He says it will make life easier for you. I believe I can vouch for that. Life is hard, but it's less hard if we let God take charge.

In the past week, I've been able to drive again. I've been out to lunch with friends and have started up the Fall Season of RCIA as a sponsor for a wonderful, young physician who wants to become a member of the Catholic Church. We meet once a week on Tuesday evenings, and I think I look forward to this faith sharing time as much as the new-to-the-Catholic-Church group. We have a big class this year, lots of camaraderie, fun, and fellowship.

Speaking of class, Christine and I have signed up together for an adult education, evening class on developing writing skills. It's taught by Herb Benham, a columnist for the local Bakersfield Californian newspaper, who is a relaxed, cool, and experienced writer. Last week he asked what we like to write. I said "Letters."

He said, "Well, you can bring some of your letters to me and I will help you edit them." (If my letters start getting shorter, you'll know why!) So now I am trying to find some of my old letters of chapter length and begin compiling them into an organized book.

I won't have time next week to do much writing because I am flying to Chicago. My niece, Gina, and her honey, Jeff, are getting married on Saturday, October 5. I've been asked to read at their wedding Mass. They have chosen the reading from Paul's letter from 1 Corinthians 13 where he speaks so vividly about Love. This is a lovely time for me to ponder that most lasting of all gifts—Love. I've seen it in you, especially these past several weeks as I've recovered from surgery. Thank you for keeping the love of God always alive through your thoughtfulness and prayers.

I love you!!!!

Nov. 2003

FAMILY LOVE

This is probably the last thing that Mimi ever wrote.

A month ago, I wasn't thinking as well as I needed to. That was a sad day! Sort of out-of-the-blue, I lost much of my ability to articulate what I was trying to say. I was scared and didn't know what was happening. Fortunately, I was at my oncologist's office, and he recognized what the problem might be. He sent me immediately for an MRI of my head.

The exam revealed what appeared to be a metastatic brain tumor right up near the front of my head, with some other areas of concern along the back in the occipital lobe. The very next day, I had an appointment with the same brain surgeon who operated on my head nine years ago. He's the best in town, and he performed surgery the very next morning . . . before I even had much time to think about it. That's probably the best way to do brain surgery . . . or probably any surgery for that matter!

What I remember most of my two days before surgery is that all my kids lovingly came home to be with me. Liz was with me through the whole doctor's appointment and MRI. She's been my driver recently and is sweet, calm, cool, and together. David, who had just been here visiting the weekend before, turned right around and came back again. He's our night owl, so he came and stayed with me at the hospital. He makes a great nurse and was extremely patient and helpful to me as I tried hard to vocalize the words I was trying to say. Robin came to visit, too, and was also very encouraging and helpful. Katie and Jeff showed up, too, despite the fact that Katie was in the midst of final study to pass her pediatric board exam, which was in five days. She managed to get back to Los Angeles for two gruesome days of a six-hour exam. Her resilience amazes me. I think Jeff provides a calming influence. He is a wonderful, compassionate person. It's easy to see why their relationship turned into love. The wedding is planned for March 13.

Christine, who probably has more friends in Bakersfield than Tony and I put together, has called upon them to help us with meals. On the day I was diagnosed with the brain tumor, she appealed to her 70-member church choir . . . and they responded way beyond anything I would have hoped. Three days a week, they bring delicious, nutritious meals. I'm going to work—putting back the weight I lost . . . and the most wonderful advantage is that I am able to spend more time relaxing and recovering while these sweet people I don't even know take time to love and care. I must say the experience has been a true Christian experience of love. It makes me want to be more useful to others when I recover.

I can't say enough about my darling Tony who has been a rock through this whole thing. He's been by my side—sheltering, encouraging, organizing, and working each day. He is a rather amazing man. In addition, he has been orchestrating a complete repainting inside and outside of our house. We're almost finished, and now we're just waiting for the new carpet. Needless to say, it's been a project we wouldn't have begun if we knew all this brain tumor shock was about to happen . . . but who knew????

Special thanks to my darling sister-in-law, Kathy, from Chicago who was on a plane out here two days after I left the hospital. She's a fabulous mother to her own four daughters . . . and Tony knew she could come and mother our kids too. All four of the kids needed her loving care and encouragement. They got plenty of it. She made homemade chicken soup, chicken divan, baked apples, and cookies. She gave love and encouragement, received love, and helped us pack up to get ready for the painters . . . in short, she went well beyond the call of duty. I don't know what I would have done without her. She surely made a difficult time easier. Just witnessing her sweet spirit made my brain feel more at ease. Her darling daughters sent surprises, which made me laugh.

There is just nothing quite like loving family and friends. Thank you so much to each of you for your concern, prayers, and love.

God has blessed me with so many loving experiences. Truly that's what I remember. In fact, I went to a retreat at our church. The retreat master cautioned us not to limit what God can do in our lives. Let God be God and allow Him to do what He wants with our lives. I intend to do that.

CHAPTER 2

Mimi's Background

I had the privilege of calling Mimi my friend for over 44 years. We met the very first day of fourth grade and remained friends for the rest of Mimi's life. She had an infectious smile and a wonderful laugh; just being with Mimi always made me feel good!

We went through nine years of school together. During our years at Trinity High School in River Forest, Illinois, we both became officers of a Club, which was the athletic organization. Mim was a swimmer and I played basketball. When we were not at our own games or meets, we were always cheering each other on to victory. It was during these years that I realized what a great cheerleader Mim was. She always gave 100 percent of her time and talents to help her friends through all types of high school crises!

In fall of 1967, Mim left Oak Park to attend Marquette University to become a physical therapist, while I stayed in Chicago to attend Loyola. It was very hard for both of us to say good-by that evening before she left. We had become so use to seeing each other every day and spending hours on the phone every night. Mim loved Marquette and soon found the love of her life, Tony Deeths. Mim and Tony were married at the end of her sophomore year and moved to Los Angeles for Tony's internship.

It was during those years that our friendship took on a whole new dynamic; we both realized that distance was never going to be an obstacle to either of us. Letters were exchanged frequently and the stock in the local phone companies continued to rise—thanks to us.

Mimi always told me that her children were God's greatest gift to her. We often spoke about our kids and hoped that they would be lucky enough to have a friendship like ours. We certainly shared many laughs over the years.

It was during her remarkable battle with cancer that I was privileged enough to share her fears and her tears. Her fears were never long lasting because of her great faith in God, and her tears were never for herself but for her family and friends. She wanted us to know how much she loved her God and us. During our last phone conversation,

Mim was quite weak but very eager to give me the latest scoop on all the Deeths.

Before I could ask her how she was doing, she wanted to know how I was. When I finally asked Mimi how she was, she answered, "I'm a little tired, but I'm still going to fight the cancer."

Mimi died about three weeks later.

Our friendship is a gift that I will always treasure! I had a friend who was loving, courageous, caring, and funny. She was a tower of strength and a fierce fighter. She taught us all that if we, as ordinary people, have faith in God, we would all be winners! Mimi, thanks for being my friend.

Triss Meyer
Mimi's long time friend

Early 1998

ALL MY ANGELS

This gives us insight into who Mimi was, how she became who she was. It also gives a history of her life and why she wanted to write a book.

Dear M. J.,

Thanks for the awesome presentation you delivered at St. Philips last weekend. I spoke to you briefly afterwards and told you to remember me (MCDeeths from CLASS Chats aol.com on Tuesdays). I said I was going to write you my story because you brought out so much of the base of my iceberg as I sat and listened to you on Saturday. I've been working with a psychologist for six months to try and figure things out. It's been hard work and exhausting but also very satisfying in many ways. To backtrack a bit, I've always been sort of an amateur psychologist, have taken a few courses, but not had much formal training. Since I've been meeting with this psychologist, it's like I can feel new circuits developing in my brain. It's a high kind of feeling. I was encouraged that you got your degrees in psychology after you had accomplished many life experience credit years. It made me realize that at 48, it's not too late for me to pursue a new interest. I'm not sure I care about the degrees, but I like the thought of the mental stimulation.

I liked what you said about the satisfaction you get from presenting your seminars and workshops—you want to share what you have learned in the hopes of helping some of us take shortcuts by identifying and rerouting certain personal villains or characteristics, which may be harmful in our relationships. You sparked many areas that I need to become more aware of in order to help myself and my family. Furthermore, you did it in such a delightfully humorous though heartfelt way that I was able to absorb it with relative ease. I listened to your tape on villains twice more the very afternoon of the seminar—and was equally entertained each time. Thank you for your gift of presentation, humor, honesty, sincerity, and love, which comes from God.

I'm trying to write a book, which is how I got tied into Marita's CLASS Chats. I am not too compulsive about that right now. It's been a three-year effort so far . . . and I am coming to realize that perhaps the process of writing is more important than the effort to get it published. If God wants it in print, He'll let me know "if" and when.

As I write this, I am helping myself solidify my thoughts. If I ramble, I'm sorry. I could identify with your villains. My mother is a Betty Blamer. That's how I grew up. She loved me, but I seldom looked right, thought right, or did what "she would have done at my age." Fortunately, I think I was born a Golden Retriever, so I tried to be good so everything would be harmonious in our family of six siblings. I don't think my dad had any villains. He was my ideal.

I grew up being a combination of a Betty Blamer and a Patsy Placater who also had the Pressure cooker personality but seldom opened the steam vent. I took pride in my Placater personality and tried to model my father's exemplary behavior. I married at the age of 20 into a whole family of Karl Computers. My husband is a radiologist who loves to look for details in X-rays, does intense stamp collecting and model ship building for relaxation, and plans his summer garden in his head all winter long. We had four children in a six-year span (now they are 20, 22, 24, and 26), and he never changed a diaper but once with our fourth child. He took pride in the fact that he interacted more than the average of 37 seconds each day with his children when they were young. (He heard that statistic on a radio talk show one day while driving to work, and that absolved him of any guilt I might have tried to lay on him concerning the subject.)

I did not find it hard to care for my children full-time. I've always loved children, and yes, I would die for mine. My husband provided for our financial needs very adequately. It was hard to play both super mom and super wife. Guess which one suffered? You know, the squeaky wheels get the oil. The kids demanded attention; my husband had plenty of solitary distractions—TV, reading, stamps, shipbuilding, gardening, building soap box derby cars with our son, and setting up science fair projects with the kids. My husband enjoyed the kids as they got to be teenagers. He liked to teach them all he knew in the Carl Computer manner. God blessed us with very good kids—they loved and respected both of us. I think I was a pretty good mom. God blessed me in that respect. I was happy in my role as mother, community volunteer, Girl Scout leader, Cub Scout leader, team mom, PTA President, etc. My husband of 27 years has always loved me and been faithful.

Six years ago, we moved from the home we had lived in for seventeen years in Missouri and settled in Bakersfield, California. My husband had a promising, new job in the land of warmth and sunshine where he had lived as a boy. He was happy. The kids took the move with their characteristic maturity. I was so proud of them. One daughter stayed behind to complete medical school in Missouri. I know it was hard for her to be separated from the rest of the family. Our second daughter left for college in San Diego that year. After some initial adjustments, our high school son and daughter settled in well and so did my husband and I. The pace of my life was the quietest that I can ever remember. I had left my friends, had only two kids left at home, and I had time on my hands so I did something I had dreamed of doing ever since I married and quit school at the age of 20—I went back to college. I loved the feeling of aged wisdom on the college campus. I met some friends my age. Speaking of age—I was beginning to feel it! My back bothered me so I decided to consult an orthopedic surgeon for a scoliosis that I had been ignoring for 25 years.

At the age of 43, I left school again—this time for extensive back surgery consisting of seven disk fusions, installing metal rods in my spine, and necessitating wearing a back brace for a year. The surgery was a biggie, but I was so proud to have faced that demon head-on after 25 years of worrying about it. That recovery was really quite relatively simple. I felt good though I tired easily. I went back to college within the year, and I stayed involved on the edges of my two high-schoolers' activities. I still felt like the "Mom" to all four of my adult children and was savoring having these two youngest high-schoolers at home. Our daily family of four was quite manageable. My husband seemed very happy and was becoming mellower in this new job situation. It was nice to see him relatively relaxed. He loved tending to his garden and landscaping in this land of lush growth, California. He and our son shared a love of computer fascination, and their whole male bonding thing was a source of great pleasure to me. I followed my daughter through varsity basketball and enjoyed the team camaraderie. Our two daughters away at college seemed happy and called regularly. I felt that we as parents deserved to lay back and sort of rest on our laurels. I felt we had earned this period of relaxation and satisfaction. We'd been married for 24 years, and God had been very good to us, more than kind, I used to say to myself . . . and smile inside.

I realized that I was smiling inside less and less lately toward the spring of 1994. Concerned, I consulted my internist. I talked to her of stress, empty nest as our son was preparing to graduate from high school, pre-menopausal symptoms, diarrhea, minor side effects from back surgery eighteen months ago, and unexplained exhaustion.

In June of that year, my worst fear was revealed to me. Many diagnostic tests, a colonoscopy, and abdominal surgery revealed that at the age of 44, I had colon cancer with involvement in the nodes and metastases to my liver. My husband and two kids at home were by my bedside from the beginning, our oldest daughter took leave of absence from medical school and flew home from Missouri immediately, our second daughter postponed plans for a big time celebration of her twenty-first birthday at school, and she came home instead to be with me.

I will digress here for a moment—remember above when I said I would die for my kids. Well, in this hospital moment I changed my mind! I knew that God had given me this husband and those kids, and I fought to live for them then, and I will continue the fight! What I have only recently learned is that my cancer was so advanced at the time of diagnosis that my family came to my side, preparing as best they could, to help me die should that become necessary. What I have also recently learned is that for three years my husband never told me the severity of my initial prognosis nor did my kids ever discuss it with me. When I discussed it recently with one of my daughters, she cried when she told me how hard it had been to hold such a painful reality in her heart. I asked her why she never brought it up so we could have talked about it. She answered, "Because, Mom, you didn't know, but you had such faith . . . and I would never take your hope away." How do you respond when in an instant you realize that you have taught a child EVERYTHING that you ever wanted to teach a kid about Love? Moments like this can only be described as presents wrapped and delivered by one of God's angels. In this case, it was my child.

There have been many angels sent by God into my life, especially since my cancer diagnosis. I won't go into them all here—that's a whole other mental vacation into God's Grace. I'll save it for another day. No, I'll save it for everyday . . . because I know His grace is there everyday.

In the past three and a half years, my husband, my children, my family, my friends, my priests, my doctors, my nurses, my psychologist—all my angels—have walked beside me through over 150 chemotherapy intravenous treatments, two abdominal surgeries, brain surgery, liver surgery, adrenal tumor surgery, two angiographic procedures, hours of MRI's and CT scans, and one ten-day hospitalization for what I can only describe as total body and brain failure. (I don't remember much about it!)

I get puzzled and confused sometimes. I become worried and anxious when I see no end in sight to the chemotherapy, which is still ongoing. My imagination allows itself to entertain frightening demons that threaten to overwhelm my sense of well-being. Alas, I still retain my pressure cooker personality and sometimes the steam has to escape. Can you imagine how that scares people—they don't know if I'm being dramatic or dying? I don't either. It's hard to be a Patsy Placator when I know that my condition is the cause of many people's concern and pain. How can I be a Betty Blamer, when in my desperate and distressing condition, I have never known anything but love and unconditional support? I never expected this condition for myself, but God obviously planned the Mystical Body resources He has provided so generously for me.

God planned? Oh my, does that make Him a Carl Computer? Meticulous planning, down to the details, seldom yells, well-educated, reasonable. . . . .or is He a Barney Blamer . . . creates fear, encourages obedience, and notices what's not done (small transgressions lead to larger ones)? Could He be a Peter Placator . . . hurting when things don't go smoothly, wanting people to work together, and feeling responsible for the pain of others? (In this life we will suffer for His sake.) Sometimes, He even seems like a Danny Distractor . . . when He doesn't answer our questions or concerns immediately, but He is a very busy God. After all, He's got a very big job watching over the world and all the people in it. How would you like to feed, clothe, and watch over all those people?

As you can tell, M.J., I am getting distracted, and it is getting late. I didn't mean to put those titles in the above paragraph to God. . . . but in doing that I came to realize that none of the villains are all bad. In fact, each of the four has some very enduring qualities, God-like qualities. It's only when we fail to recognize and control the dark side that hurts others that we are weakened, and they become villains in our lives. Thank you for making me more aware of the power I possess, with the grace of God, to control my attitudes and reactions. You have been a great contributor to my psychotherapy, perhaps speeding my reaction time and my recovery . . . Thanks for being an enzyme!

I will keep your husband in my prayers along with other fellow cancer survivors. I empathize with his frustration with exhaustion. I pray that we will learn more to be accepting like Paul who stated than "when I am weak, then I am strong." May all your future endeavors be successful—I hope your husband will soon be able to accompany you once again in your speaking ministry.

With love and prayers for you and your family,

Early 1999

A PHLEGMATIC LOOKS BACK AND
MOVES FORWARD . . .

*Mimi went to a conference once on the four major personal-
ity types. After the class, she decided to write the story. It gives us
a good understanding of how she became the person she was.*

Growing up as a quiet and somewhat shy phlegmatic was a
good place to be. I was the middle child in a family of four brothers.
My only little sister was set apart from the rest of us five by an age
span of four years. She was definitely the "baby" of the family and far
too protected to enter into the scheming of us older five. We five were
bonded by being born in a five-year age span from start to finish. Mom
was content to take care of baby Suzie while the rest of us went off into
our fantasy playtime.

The boys shared a dormitory-type room with double bunk beds
while I got to have a room of my own. When the pressure of competi-
tion got too much for one of the guys to handle, they would come into
my room for respite time. I got to know each of them as an individual,
whereas the rest of the world saw them only as "those Davy boys."
They were a rowdy, restless bunch of guys with boundless energy and
a spirit of competitive one-upmanship with each other that resulted in
a lot of foolish and funny antics around our house.

Our dad, the phlegmatic father, would sit back, relaxed, and
smile at his silly sons. I liked to do that too. My mom, the powerful
choleric, tried to tame them by lecturing endlessly on manners and setting schedules and threatening punishments if she found out they were
not complying. One threat was that she was going to tell dad when he
got home from work. We all giggled secretly about that one because we
knew dad would not be mad at us but would simply spend his time
trying to settle my mom's nerves down. The boys took delight in getting her stirred up. One of my favorite frequently repeated scenes was
to watch mom, out of sheer frustration, chase one of the boys around
the house with her broom when she had her fill of his foolishness. The
race continued until she got so exhausted that she had to quit. Looking
back, I think that was a great form of stress release for her, and I'm not
sure she would actually have hit one of her boys even if she had come
within swiping distance!

I loved my funny brothers. They were like a Four Stooges movie playing endlessly before me, and I was quite content to watch. They were no threat to me, and I did not interfere with their lives unless they asked me to. I considered their requests the supreme flattery. When they had homework they needed help with, girlfriend problems to discuss, money needed for a movie, or minor infractions they needed help covering up, they knew they could come to me for sanctuary. I didn't mind at all for they added a certain spice to my quiet kind of life.

As I grew into my teens, I tried to become more like my brothers. I tried to be a vibrant personality, I tried to be wild. I tried to bounce off people the way they did. I failed. I remained the serious, shy, studious, servant-type, and I was content with that. Surprisingly, somewhere around my junior year in high school, people started to notice me. I was asked to join clubs; I was chosen for the volleyball team. I was nominated for vice president. This sudden popularity surprised me, and I questioned people how it all happened. People said it was because I got along with EVERYBODY. Phlegmatics tend not to irritate anybody nor get too bothered by what others do, and I do believe that is somewhat unusual as a teenager. Thus I stood out amongst my peers as the even tempered, ever consistent one.

I realized I got along with everybody, but it wasn't because I went out of my way to notice them or to be nice. I just had an easy time accepting them for who they were—people didn't irk me because I happen to be a personality that is not easily irked! Nevertheless, I was forced into a more public role. It felt good to be sought out, and I dutifully carried out the high school and college roles expected of me. I learned as an adult, however, that I was not good at saying "No" to other's seemingly endless requests for volunteer help.

After marriage and the births of our four children, I was a "nonworking" mother. In an era where the feminist movement was challenging many young moms to go back to the workplace, I was left as the logical choice for filling all sorts of volunteer positions. Somehow, I got to believing that the world wouldn't keep revolving if I didn't help it out. I was not having fun being chairman and volunteer coordinator for everything from Girl Scout cookie chairman to PTA president. I would work too hard—I didn't know how to ask for help, too shy to bother "busy" others, and definitely not assertive enough to speak out. Then I would feel upset because I didn't think I was doing the job as well as I could have.

The experience, however, turned out to be valuable. Although it was a lot of work, I did come to realize that I as a more public personality, people come to know you, trust you, and seek out your advice. I began to see that no one expected me to do everything, but they did appreciate what I had done and came to me sort of as a consultant when they had to deal with some of the obstacles I had dealt with.

In many ways I felt as if I had come full circle. From a shy child, to an involved teenager and adult, and then back to a quieter and wiser more mature adult. I was able to look back, see my areas of disquietude in large group social inadequacy, and move forward into the place God planned my personality to move.

In college I had studied physical therapy because it was an area where I could be helping people in a one-on-one working situation. As a young mother with four young children, I was often asked by other mothers how I managed with my family; Motherhood was my proudest occupation, and I was definitely in my comfort zone as I talked to new young mothers and explained to them all you basically needed to do was love those babies, the rest followed. My children turned out to be serious, bright, motivated students—largely from the patient influence of their father—and again people would ask me how I did it. I could tell them honestly that I didn't do much. I said that they had their father's "smart" genes, and I was content to just let them grow and develop into who they wanted to be.

For a phlegmatic personality that is pretty easy. They grew into an interesting cadre of four, and I derived the same delight watching them as I had watching my brother's years earlier. They came to me when they needed help or advice. I was happy to give it, though it often went ignored. As is often the case, children work through their own problems oftentimes just by talking about them with someone who will listen. I had always been good at listening. Meantime, they put their own creative personality decisions toward the solution, and they would be satisfied with that.

I hope you are getting the drift of who I am. I like doing things for others—it suits me far better than being in charge of others. Looking back, there were definitely times when I could have used a bit more of an outgoing nature. I was sometimes embarrassed by my shyness and my quiet way of accepting things, but God knows the plan He has for each of us. Now I am coming to realize that my quiet acceptance serves me well. Five years ago, I was stunned by the news that I had inoperable cancer. My prognosis was not at all promising. I was never good at talking so I didn't talk about my disease. The doctors talked about it. My husband and grown children talked about it while I slept easily under the influence of morphine. Sleeping, after all, is one of a phlegmatic's greatest moments of peace.

The sleep allowed my body to recover from the onslaught of the surgeon's tools. The oncologist felt that since I was relatively young and recovering well, I was a healthy candidate for some experimental treatment. He approached me with his plan. My husband gave his consent. My kids thought it was my best hope. I thought it was great—the people I love most had made my decision for me! All I had to do was follow along . . .

I have followed their advice for nearly five years now. I have yet to enter the remission phase of my disease, and so I remain on weekly chemotherapy. That's sickening, and it forces me to remain quiet several days each week, but I am moving forward with my life. I am moving forward with discovering more about myself in my quiet retreat. I am finding God because I have time to listen for His voice. I am not shy with Him. He is much like me. I love His phlegmatic, quiet acceptance of who I am!

Sept. 2002

MY NAME IS MIMI

Mimi took a writing class with her daughter Christine from a local columnist in 2002. The first assignment was to write a short story on "Who am I?"

"How did you get that name?" people often asked.

My answer is that it was by default. On the day my mom and dad brought their baby girl named Mary Catherine home from the hospital, my two brothers, ages 1 and 2, couldn't pronounce such a mouthful of a name. They called me Mimi. So did everyone else.

I had a wonderful, relatively carefree childhood during the early years of the post-World War Baby Boom. Mom was a hard worker, always busy cleaning and cooking for our three generational household, which soon numbered ten. Mom didn't have a lot of time for fun, but dad liked to play. When he got home from work, Mom always said, "Take these kids and let them run off steam so they'll calm down. We showed dad all the tricks we learned that day on the swing set in the yard. He always laughed at us. I couldn't believe what a nice arrangement that was. Mom, the strict one, was inside cooking dinner while dad, the playmate, was out in the backyard with us!

I had a wonderful and relatively carefree childhood, growing up in Chicago. I was surrounded by a large, Irish extended family, lots of kissing and hugging, and cousins to play with. I was spoiled by my Gramma Nana who lived with us. She would walk with me to the soda fountain in the drugstore across the street. Sometimes, we'd ride the village bus to town for shopping. The boys usually didn't get to go. Gramma Nana thought they were too wild. I couldn't believe how lucky I was to have such a Nana!

I was a quiet child, big for my age and strong. Since Mom wanted us to burn off steam, we kids walked to the swimming pool every day in the summer. My task there was to learn to swim as fast as I could so I could escape being caught and dunked underwater by my two older, rambunctious brothers. I helped teach my two little brothers and my sister to swim and protected them from any bullies that came along. Both my speed and lesson-giving experience paid off. I joined the competitive swim team and was a member of the relay team, which set the Illinois state record when I was twelve. During my high school summers, I made money as a lifeguard and swimming instructor at the big, new, Olympic size swimming pool, which had just been completed in our village. How lucky I was to get that for a first job!

Because of my athletic ability and my interest and curiosity about medical things, I chose to major in physical therapy in college. I was accepted at Marquette University in Wisconsin and loved the experience of living in a dorm for three years. By the end of my junior year, I had traded in dorm life for wife life. Eleven months later, instead of a degree in my hand, I held our first baby in my arms. I've never really regretted the change in plans.

Within the next six years, my husband Tony and I had added three more children to our family. Those were busy years but very satisfying ones. I considered myself very fortunate to be a stay-at-home mother because I loved to be involved in the lives of my husband and children. I didn't keep a Martha Stewart home, but I focused instead on the fun and delight of the children's creativity. When the kids went off to school, I went with them. I worked in the library, as room mother, Brownie leader, Cub Scout leader, Girl Scout leader, and as PTA co-president, I helped establish a publishing house at the elementary school where the kids could come with their ideas and get some adult help with their writing. That was probably the most satisfying role I had in all my volunteer years.

Sept. 2002

WHY I AM TAKING THE WRITING CLASS TAUGHT BY HERB BENHAM

This was written during the class Mimi took with Herb.
It gives insight into why she loves writing.

I like to write letters and send them because I think I am able to better express my feelings in a letter than in quickly spoken words. A well-written letter gives me a sense of pride not unlike what a craftsman must feel after finishing a custom piece of furniture. A piece of pretty paper written upon with a pen or an attractive computer font can bring a lost art alive. I like to think of myself as an artist. I'm taking this class so I will improve my skills.

I remember once watching a furniture maker in a tourist turn of the century town creating a piece of quality furniture. I marveled at the repetitive strokes and the aura of patient relaxation the craftsman exhibited. As the shape of a chair leg became apparent, the block of wood had developed a life of its own. As the project progressed, a complete chair took shape and the finished piece provided a place to sit and rest. That's what I like about letter writing. Repetitive strokes of my hands create words, and soon the letter has taken on a life of its own. My thoughts have created it, and those thoughts will soon provide enjoyment for the person who will sit and rest and read it.

Letter writing is one way I have of relieving stress. I can relax when I am doing repetitive tasks with no deadline. Creativity can blossom. I feel smart, alive, and more in control as the project unfolds and begins to move along smoothly. In this easily flowing part of the letter, I begin to reveal who I am, how I am feeling, and why I am writing to this particular person. In revealing why I am writing to you, I come to love and appreciate you more. I realize how my life has been enriched because of my relationship with you.

A letter can make both me and the receiver feel good. I view my letter as a gift to the person and intend that it will brighten the day and be will received with appreciation, and perhaps, gratitude. Over my lifetime of letter writing, I've had several people tell me that they were moved by something I wrote. This encourages me to continue writing. Sometimes if I write a long letter full of timely information, I will make a copy and save it to serve as my own memory bank.

Many of my letters are personal anecdotes or family stories. Others are more like private diary or journal entries. Some are nearly book chapter length.

Frequently, I find my jotted notes among my house clutter and sit down and read about thought, feelings, or events that may have happened months or even years ago. It's like reliving a dream, but the concrete writing reminds me that the dream was real. I like to remember and reassemble the events end emotions, which tell the story that is my life.

I'm taking this class because I lack the discipline to organize my writing, but I want to compile my scribbles and stories. I intend to use this class as an anchor to hold me bound to that purpose. I want to leave here and go home with the desire to open dusty drawers, comb through closet shelves, and plow through piles of random papers to find those precious memories and reminders. I want to assemble them in a notebook and create a book. I don't care to market it or to publish it. I just want to take it over to Kinkos, copy it, and give a copy to my kids . . .

Oh that finished project will make me feel organized. What an inspiration this class will have been if that happens!

CHAPTER 3

More History

I knew Mimi Deeths B.C. (Before Cancer) when we both lived in St. Louis. She was always special.

Throughout Mimi's cancer struggle, she was a fighter—from the first surgery through all the nearly 10 years of other surgeries and treatments. After diagnosis, a group of St. Louis friends decided to visit her. Although her cancer was extensive, we had a lot of fun together. After we left, she learned she had a massive brain tumor. It continued . . .

Through the years, we had multiple traveling adventures. The years saw Mimi getting progressively weaker. Cancer, along with the treatments, was taking a toll on her body, but it never robbed her of her joyous spirit. Our group knew Mimi BEFORE cancer—and that was an important distinction to her.

Everyone was affected by Mimi—by who she was, by her struggles, by her faith, by her generosity, by her gift of herself to everyone. When my sister's cancer reactivated, Mimi called her in support. Although Mimi herself was battling, she was always reaching out to others at the same time. Talking to her—one could never tell that she was ill; she was always full of life and vitality—and fun! Hope sprang eternal.

Her ability to battle cancer for such a long time was just amazing—but mostly it was her attitude. She maintained cheerfulness and faith while very ill from the treatments. She was able to counsel cancer patients and to give them the courage and strength to continue with their own treatments. She inspired all of us.

I have said, "Mimi accomplished so much while dealing with cancer; I can only imagine what she could have accomplished had she been well." However, I think some of her accomplishments were due to her cancer—the chemo patients she touched, the faith-filled letters she wrote. She touched so many people in her 54 short years; it is impossible to have known her and not have been affected by this incredible person. I know Mimi would think that cancer was a gift given to her by God. If God wants us to use our gifts wisely, then He is most pleased with Mimi.

The last time I spoke with her, she was in hospice; everyone knew the end was near. Her voice was so full of excitement about her daughter's wedding, it was difficult to accept what I knew to be true. When I told Mimi she sounded great, she said she was not certain if she should give up the fight. But she also told me how she was struggling to find the right words to say to each of her children—because she knew too.

How typical Mimi that was . . . at the very end she was concerned about her family. It speaks to her whole life. I miss her dearly—her wisdom—her laughter. How blessed I am to be her friend.

Betty Serati
Mimi's friend and member of playgroup
October 13, 2004

Feb. 1998

REFLECTING BACK

This letter is a good summary of Mimi's years with cancer.

February 18, 1998

Dear Faye and Jim,

I was so happy to hear your message on the recorder. Thanks for being such a caring and thoughtful friend. I'm sorry for my lack of consideration. We left many of our good friends hanging this Christmas, and I still feel very badly about that . . . but neither Tony nor I have had the initiative to get going with our Christmas list letters.

You are right about your comment that my voice sounds good. Physically I seem to be doing well. My mental emotional state has left something to be desired for the past six months or so. I know you can understand.

To back track a bit—the problem seems to have begun last June (7 months ago). I flew to Chicago to visit my mom who at the age of 78 had brain aneurysm surgery. As she was recovering from that, she suffered a ruptured appendix and had a second emergency surgery within a month. She was physically recovering well, but she had some anxiety attacks while I was there. She can't deal with my illness, let alone her own. At the same time my mother was failing, Tony's dad entered into the final stages of Alzheimer's and no longer knew who his wife of 63 years. He began to require full-time nursing assistance. It has been difficult for Tony and me to deal with the emotional needs of three aging parents. Tony's mom and dad live about 1 1/2 hours from us, and Tony spends most evenings on the phone encouraging his mom. Tony's older brother (at the age of 60) was diagnosed with prostate cancer and had a heart attack several months later. He is doing all right now but has had to nearly retire from his urology practice.

In addition to dealing with our older family members, we had the kids in and out for vacations this summer. In talking with them, we came to realize that they have some emotional needs largely resulting from my cancer diagnosis. I have chosen to rely on my faith and try to take one day at a time. I have never gone back to face what happened when I was initially diagnosed. I did not want to and probably was unable to because of the location of my brain tumor (in the brain area of emotion and higher level thinking, found and removed 5 months after diagnosis). Anyway, when I realized the kids' (and Tony's) needs, I began to open myself to listen to their problems dealing with my cancer diagnosis. This was an incredibly emotional family exercise.

What I perhaps realized but never acknowledged was that at the time of my diagnosis, my internist and surgeon told my family that I had perhaps two weeks to several months to live. My oncologist has confirmed that my prognosis was "poor," but because of my otherwise good health, my faith, and my support system, and relatively young age, he was willing to attempt some unusual medical interventions (hepatic catheter with a 24-hour chemo drip to attack the colon mets in my liver). All I was ever aware of was the success of my treatment and the hand of God constantly present. My family did not fully enter into this faith journey with me, and they still try to cope with that diagnosis.

Well, Faye and Jim, you well know that when someone you love is hurting, you bear some of their pain. I took on the pain of my family members and began to wake-up nights thinking I had only weeks to live. It was my own going back to the beginning and sorting things out in my mind. I have been seeing a professional therapist (also a cancer survivor) since July . . . and actually, it has taken me on a most fascinating journey through the power of the mind and relationships with others. It does, however, require an incredible amount of hard work. I feel like I am dissecting my head and those of my family. I am exhausted much of the time. My nerves were ragged frequently.

Contributing to this problem is the fact that 3 1/2 years after my original diagnosis, I still remain on 5-FU chemo. It is doing its own job on my nerves . . . so I can never tell if the problem is physical or mental. We've decided it is a combination of both. The physical effects most likely cause increased mental agitation. Throw in a few hormonal problems like chemo wiping out my ovary, one adrenal removed for metastases, and all the other organs and glands subjected to 5-FU . . . and the picture becomes a bit more complicated.

Interestingly enough, we are studying the letters of Paul in Bible Study Fellowship, and that is contributing greatly to my attitude adjustment. He finds joy and purpose in his trials. I am trying to do the same in mine. I have a great support system.

My oncologist is very helpful, and he is trying to keep track of all aspects of my treatment. This is how chemo is going: Last August (1997) I completed three nonstop years of 5-FU and Leukovorin. It had been a full year since the last metastaic surgery, which was in my left adrenal gland. My CEA was averaging about 3.5 for that year. My oncologist and I decided to wean slowly off chemo and not just stop it abruptly. I switched from weekly IV to every other week in August.

I liked the alternate week therapy because I could actually have a normal healthy full week in between the "side effect week." However, my CEA began to climb almost immediately. It went to 4, then 5, then 6, then 5.5 (that showed promise) then it went to 7, then to 10. Right now it remains at 10.2. I was going berserk! The uncertainty began to drive me nuts. It still does, but I am coping better in these past few weeks.

You might guess that I was not coping well at Christmastime. In fact, I entered the Christmas season on a very sour note. In September, Tony lost his job. He handled the entire situation in a manner that made me proud. He was very gentlemanly about it, but I let anger eat at my soul. Corporate bad manners and greed of the large HMO his group serviced led to the dissolution of his radiology group's contract. The HMO had sneakily extended the contract out for bids to four other radiology groups in the area, the whole time telling Tony and his partner that they were entirely pleased with their services (eight years of good service). We believe the other radiology group of 16 doctors was able to come in low bid or capitation and defeat Tony's small group of 2. I know that is big business; what makes me mad is that it all comes down to money. With many HMO's—cheap medicine means "best." I felt very emotional about this and tied it into my situation. Had I been insured by that HMO, I would be dead now because they would not have put their money into a "terminal" case. I am trying hard not to harbor grudge—God has a master plan.

I need to keep that focus on God. Thanks to your many ministry tapes, Faye, I have been helped in keeping that focus. Originally when you sent them, I did not find time to listen to very many of them. I kept them filed for easy reference on a rainy day. The "rainy" days came, but actually they were lovely sunny days, and I started to relieve my stress and anger by long walks in the neighborhood complete with headphones and your tapes. It is hard to be frustrated and angry when one is listening to people like Leo Buscaglia and those other retreat masters while enjoying a beautiful day.

I think of you often, and thank you for the gift you sent to me way last year. Those tapes brighten many a day. Even in your absence, you minister to me. I hope you and Jim and the girls are happy and healthy. I promise I'll try to do a better job corresponding. Thank you for your sweet surprise phone message—it affirmed once again how many people care. You are an angel (Hebrew 1: 13–14). God bless you.

Mid-2001

OVERWHELMED

This is an update letter Mimi wrote after her birthday in 2001.

June 25 was my birthday—actually my birthday started several days before that. A few of my very organized friends had cards in the mail the week before. Some others talked about, 'Let's do lunch for your birthday' . . . Oh, my goodness! How could I fit in a birthday??

Birthday, birthdays, why celebrate birthdays anyway? " I don't need any special days. Everyday is "special" I would say. Besides, I'm still sending thank-you's for my fiftieth—that was two years ago! Let me catch up with that one, please . . . don't pile on anymore!

The days just prior to my birthday this year were busy ones. I had taken on a most delightful summer project—playing "teacher" to my little triplet 6- year-old friends. Riley, Samantha, and Zachary had been coming over each morning for "summer-time school" where we sat at the kitchen table and practiced first grade skills, allowing for distractions and silly stories, feeding my new fish, and, of course, snacks. By afternoon, I was ready for a nap because as you know, I'm still on the chemotherapy minipump, which not only pumps in cancer control juice but also brain fuzzies and body fatiguers. I certainly didn't want to go to lunch and fall asleep in my plate! No birthdays, please . . .

Carolyn, Francine, Susan, and Conrad took Amparo and me out to lunch on the Friday between our two, June birthdays. The Fresh Choice restaurant was the setting for two Beta goldfish aquariums complete with bows and plants and fish food. Then we got matching, flowered, yard pennants and beautiful 20-inch high garden angel statues. It was a BIG display. Everyone in the restaurant knew it was our birthday. I also came home sporting a new silver and bronze giraffe pin . . . and I thought all weekend about how very thoughtful those friends are as I fed my fish, hung up my flying flower, found a special place for my garden angel, and wore my giraffe pin to church on Sunday. Mostly, I thought about each of those friends . . . and the special things they do for me all year round . . . and ever since I have known them . . . Thank you, God, for giving me friends like these.

My real birthday was on a Monday. I had the day planned out. I would meet with four friends at 7:00 A.M. for our weekly accountability group. This is a group of writers and motivational speakers, and we've decided to meet every Monday morning and plan our goals for the week over coffee. My goal that day was to celebrate another year . . . every day! They help remind me of that every Monday morning. After that, I would pick up the triplets at 9:30 and work with them for the morning. Then I would go to Mass at noon, and then at 2:00, I had an appointment at the Cancer Center to get a refill on my pump-pack. (Some birthday present, I thought, and then smiled as I thought again—yes, it is SOME birthday present . . . for it represents an opportunity so long as God wills for me to live.) Birthdays present a time to sit back and just recall how much I like to live.

Speaking of living . . . there was lots of liveliness when I arrived at the door of the triplet's house . . . where I could hear unusually excited whispers going on inside the house as I rang the front door bell. When the door opened, I was greeted with the four smiling faces (mom, Cindy, included) of my friends with a gift bag. The bag was incidental; the smiles were priceless. I hadn't mentioned my birthday to any of them and wondered how they knew. The answer lies in a child's idea of life's priorities. They told me that the day last week when my friend called and left an early birthday song on my answering machine, they went right home and told their mom that my birthday was coming up. When you're six years old, birthdays are milestones . . . and when you're 52 and share that day with three 6-year-olds, it's a very special celebration! Their mom gifted me with a lovely vase to put fresh flowers in and the kids said they picked the pink candle that smells so nice. Not so much for the beauty of a candle but for practical use, as Zach told me to "just keep it right out on my kitchen table so you can see it all the time and then you can light it if the power goes out." Zach likes to know that all his friends are prepared for an emergency, and birthdays are a good time to handle that stuff. Thank you, God, for the laughter and the love, the kisses, and the caring responses of little children . . . and the parents who teach them.

After saying good-bye to the triplets, I went to Mass at noon. My friend Judith, who had wanted to make arrangements prior to my birthday and get together with a group of friends for the big day, was there at Mass. A week earlier when she called to ask if there would be a good day to get together for my birthday, I told her that I did not want to commit myself to feeling good at a certain hour of a certain day during the following week. Because of the constant drip chemotherapy pump, there are days that I feel really fine and days that I feel not so fine. I said "Please, let's not **plan** a birthday celebration." Judith understood what I meant . . . and she just appeared at Mass next to me on the day of my birthday . . . and she was like another candle on God's altar in that church where God and his goodness in communion with so many friends provide the finest kind of birthday celebrations. Thank you, Holy Spirit, for strengthening my faith in God and for the loving intercessory prayers of my church community. Bill Devereaux sang a birthday song to me in the church vestibule after Mass, and the rest of the noon group joined in. Bill likes to start a ruckus; everybody else caught on. So many friends . . . every one of them set in place by a very loving God. Awesome thought isn't it? The very same God "who brings out the starry host one by one and calls them each by name . . . not one of them is missing" (Isaiah 40:26) is the very same God who arranges the paths in our lives and the people who will walk them with us. He holds us all in the palm of his hand. Thank you, God, for making me feel secure .

We went from God's house to In N' Out Burger. Transitions are an exciting part of life. There's a new one just down the street from Church. Handy, isn't it? Remember I told you my friend Judith was at church? Remember, I wrote earlier that I told Judith ' No birthday celebrations, please' the week before? Well, Judith wasn't **planning** lunch, but she wondered if I felt up to it. Now I have to be honest— even though I'm on chemotherapy and sometimes it might be hard to stay awake, I seldom have a problem with eating. Never have. I said, "Sure." I felt dressed just about right for In N' Out Burger too. I had on some new peddle pushers (those are what people, who are 52, call Capri-length pants—it makes our kids laugh). The other thing about my looks was this: Just the week before I had literally 'flipped my wig" that I had been wearing because I was a baldy for the last two years. Now I was on a new chemotherapy that I was very "attached to," liter-ally, via intravenous line and pocket pump 24 hours a day! The nice thing is this doesn't make my hair fall out so it's actually growing in. Since I live in BAKErsfield, and we literally bake here in the 100 degree summer heat, I was ready to shed that hot wig. Problem is the hair that grew in looked just like my brother Bill's hair. You know the type— imagine 1/2 inch, gray, and curly just like a sheep! I laughed at myself in the mirror every morning. Now I know where Bill gets the great sense of humor. You just look at yourself, laugh, and then learn to like it. Truly, thinking about Bill first thing every morning gave me a really uplifting start to the day! He's one of those guys who goes through life armed with a great sense of humor. He's handsome too. I didn't like my hair on me, but I do like it on him . . . though even he confessed that it took a lot of years of getting used to. I figured; if he could like that hair, I could too.

Anyway, to get back to the In N' Out Burger story . . . I had the peddle pushers; I had the hair, which I had put a light brown rinse on (so it looked blonde), and I had Judith who said I looked fine . . . so off we went! We honked our horn in Ginny's driveway. She was wearing her bedroom slippers in the kitchen, but when she saw our looks, she felt totally comfortable hopping in the car with her slippers on. Tina's house is on the way so we stopped to see if she was home. She was working in the yard and had mud on her pants, but she figured she fit in nicely with the three of us. We laughed all the way to In N' Out because we are grown, respectable ladies who usually try to do things very properly . . . but it was my birthday. I had blonde sheep hair . . . and since we are all old enough, we felt like we could act however we wanted. We made the young girls behind the order counter laugh . . . because laughter is so contagious. We ran into Barb Shipman who was there with her two teenage grandchildren, and they were good ones to meet to stretch out the silliness. Then the counter girls organized the birthday song at our table . . . and the face wearing the blonde sheep hair turned red—but it was one of those "freeze frame" life moments that defines the word friendship. Thank you God for friends who love me just the way I am.

I was late for my 2:00 appointment at the Cancer Center but wasn't worried about that. Nobody else wants my stuff . . . so it was just waiting there for me. Those nurses are very forgiving—even when you are late, they are just happy you're still able to come! I was there for about an hour, snoozed in the quiet, air-conditioned room, and left with a refill for another week . . . Thank you God for the doctors and nurses whose wisdom and intelligence helps improve the quality of life for others.

I drove home thinking what a busy birthday I was having. Nothing big, just lots of little things. I grabbed the mail on my way in and smiled at the familiar handwriting of my MOM. Sometimes she sends me funny cards. This year she sent a beautiful lavender card with flowers that says, "You are my daughter—my hopes and my dreams—my joy and my heart." Mothers really feel like that. I fell asleep in the chair dreaming of my mom . . . Thank you, God, for the mother you chose for me. I love her.

Ding, dong. Wake up, sleepyhead. Answer the doorbell. It's Katie! Katie had two days off and had driven up from Los Angeles to celebrate our birthdays together—hers is the day after mine. I thought about my mother's card when I saw my own daughter. My hopes and my dreams on the day she was born (28 years ago) and here she was . . . MY joy and MY heart. The other joys of my heart called from Tacoma, Lancaster, and San Diego. Thank you, God, for my grown kids who pop in and out of my life like that.

Speaking of popping in and out . . . I popped my telephone message button in . . . and got a Happy Birthday message from my sister's father-in-law, Bob McNulty, who shares the same birth date as me. Bob was born a few years before me and reminds me of a little, Irish leprechaun . . . with a gift of trickery and a heart of gold. He had open heart surgery within the same year that I was diagnosed with cancer. We CELEBRATE our birthdays because we've both been scared enough to wonder if we'd see another one. We've both felt surrounded in crisis by the love of our families and been strengthened in faith by the experience. Thank you, God, for the gift of my life . . . and all the surprises, the silences, and the sensitive moments that every birthday helps us remember.

Special surprises included a phone call from Marcia and John who were meeting their new baby granddaughter in Iowa, a phone call from Judy Honerkamp who remembers to call even when I forget to answer her letters for six months, a parking lot meeting with Mary after church when she gave me a little, and a giraffe necklace that she has had since February (now there's a gal whose got it together). Speaking of having it all together, my Aunt Mimi and Uncle Joe sent me a letter AND a birthday card marked envelope #1 and envelope #2. The Play-group girls remembered my day with cards and copies of the pictures we had taken in Las Vegas (thanks, girls, for the flattering photos—a wig, a beer, and a fake body makes me look pretty good). My little niece, Danielle, sent me an invitation to her 2-year-old birthday party and reminded me once again of her arrival in this world exactly 50 years after mine (another mutual birthday). Along with birthday celebrations for me were birth announcements from two of my nieces—Diana and Joe became first time parents to Desiree Marie, and Lisa and Joe became happy parents of their third child, Olivia Anne. Mark and Selena became parents to Mark Jacob five days after my birthday. I like to think of those little lives just beginning . . . Gifts of love and laughter and Congratulations and Happy Birthday to all of you.

Gifts, gifts, where do they all come from? Katie and I went shopping for her birthday, and we found some presents at the store. We came home laden with our gifts, and there were more outside our front door. There was a big box from my sister Sue and a heart-shaped topiary plant and a purse from Judith, who had stopped by while we were out. My birthday was supposed to be over, but late presents were extending the celebration. Stop, stop. I have already had too much birthday happiness. How can I say thank you to all these people? Then I figured not to worry about it now—just open Sue's box. Katie and I hoped there will be Fannie May candy from Chicago in it . . . and Sue has not disappointed us. We sit and savor a lavish feast of chocolate and bonbons . . . and laugh in our luxury. Good thing the Noah's Ark outfit Mark and Sue sent with the candy is a size extra-extra large! A candy for me . . . a candy for Katie . . . a candy for the giraffe . . . a candy for the monkey . . . a candy for the ox . . . a candy for the elephant . . . a candy for the pig . . . a candy for me . . . Thank you, Mark and Sue for your "sweet," thoughtful ways. My siblings and in-laws are always so thoughtful. Jeff and Lenni send a Mass card, a special remembrance . . . Thank you God for uniting us all despite the distances that separate us.

Amparo gave me stationery and special rubber stampers. Betty gave me a prayer journal with Scripture verses in it. They both know I want to write more, but I have a hard time disciplining myself to do it. Thank you, God for all the friends who encourage me . . .

Thank you for the life I have. It is indeed something to write about. My birthday is a reminder of all I have to be thankful for. I am overwhelmed by the thoughtfulness of my family and friends, the small and the big things people do for me, the Faith that I have, the miracles that have happened, and the way God has planned and provided for me in ways that I never could have imagined . . . by putting people like you in it.

I thought about all the special times I've enjoyed this summer as I fell asleep next to Tony, who had worked all through my birthday fun times. On his way home, he stopped and bought a birthday cake and cookies at the bakery. We went to dinner at our favorite Italian restaurant and talked about last week's adventure when Liz, Katie, and I had a girls' day in Los Angeles and then went to see Lion King play in Hollywood. Tony provided the theater tickets . . . happy pre-birthday to you . . . and then he bought me airline tickets so I could fly back and see Christine in Wisconsin . . . happy post-birthday to you. He works too hard, but he cares very much that his family is happy. His wisdom in medical decisions has helped keep me alive. His hard work is what provides for my comfort, my recuperation, leisure time, daily Mass, and special times with my children who've been planted now in cities scattered across the map. Thank you, God, for the husband you chose for me, and thank you for blessing our marriage the way you do.

Now you probably know more about my birthday than you ever needed to know, but I wanted to record the unique day I had and all the special people who made it so nice. I was feeling rested and well and truly able to reflect so I thought I'd get back to my writing again and thought that my birthday would be a fun topic to play with. After I began to write, I thought perhaps some of you would like to walk into a day of my life. I hope the day didn't seem to long . . .

In case you liked that day, I'll give you more highlight of the past six months. There have been good days and a few difficult ones. I know I fell behind in communicating lately. My pile of unanswered letters tells me. My intentions are good, but I usually don't get to it. However, here is a quick rundown on the highlights of this past six months:

The New Year, 2001, started with the diagnosis of another tumor, this one above my left kidney. By late February, my doctors and I decided to treat it with five weeks of daily radiation and wearing a minipump attached to me with an intravenous line delivering chemo-therapy 24 hours a day for seven weeks.

Before I began the chemotherapy and radiation, Tony and I went to a medical meeting weekend in Las Vegas. David was able to drive up from San Diego to meet us, and we had three very enjoyable days there. I was amazed by the new buildings such as the Paris Hotel, the Bellagio, we saw Circe du Soleil, and the Impressionist Art Exhibit, and we spent a nice afternoon with my niece, Julie, who lives there now.

The month of March and most of the month of April passed quickly as I slept off the side effects of the radiation. I really did not feel bad, just exhausted. I probably slept 15 to 20 hours a day after going in each morning for radiation. One weekend when I was feeling good, I drove down to Katie's apartment and then she and I went to River-side to see my brother, Bud, and Lynn and all their growing family. My brother Bob, Sue, and Brynn (from Chicago) were spending spring break in Palm Springs so they drove up to meet us for the day . . . Thank you God for the fun when family members can get together . . . even though we are all spread far and wide.

Liz was home for spring break, and Katie was able to get home for Easter weekend. We just spent time hanging around at home, but anytime when the kids are home is time to be savored . . .

By late April I was able to join Tony for five days in San Diego for a radiology meeting. David and his girlfriend, Robin, came to meet us at the hotel, and we enjoyed spending time together. David brought the new book he had authored titled *Sun Cluster Environments* . (Although it sounds like he might have done a study of popular leisure resorts (get it?) the book really is a very heavy-duty computer manual for the Sun Microsystems Corporation where he works. I like it because I am mentioned by name on the dedication page. My cousin, Gail Gardner, had us all to her house in San Diego for dinner. We heard about her months in Colorado skiing, and she filled us in on the rest of the Gardner family. We enjoyed seeing Smokey and his son. David was in a fencing tournament (sword fight) that weekend so I got to watch him fence, very well, I might add. He had just returned from Japan (business trip) a few days before our arrival in San Diego so he shared some of his adventures. It's nice knowing people who go to exciting places . . . because then it's sort of like you went there yourself . . . Thank you, God, for the beauty and assorted cultures of the world.

I met with my Saint Louis girlfriends (six of us) in Las Vegas on the first weekend in May. We try to get together every year somewhere in the United States. We always have a great time. I was a little concerned about my stamina with the Playgroup (that's what we called ourselves when we met in one another's basements when our kids were all preschoolers—so the kids could play. Now the kids are all out working—and *we* play!) I spent my last night there with my niece, Julie, and appreciated her wonderful hospitality. Thank you, God, for the wonder of watching our children grow up.

The high point of the year was Liz's graduation from University of Puget Sound. She graduated on Mother's Day (May 13) and now has a degree in occupational therapy. Tony and I and Katie and David were all able to be there to celebrate with her. We had a picnic on the riverfront the day before graduation and met all her friends. After graduation, we took Liz and her roommates out to dinner to celebrate. Katie and David could only spend the weekend in Tacoma with us, but Tony, Liz, and I spent the rest of the week touring the Upper Peninsula in Washington. The giant Sequoia forest, the rain forests, the rivers, and ocean were magnificent. Between graduation and beginning her six-month internship, Liz was able to come back to California for a couple weeks, be in a friend's wedding, spend a day in Los Angeles with Katie, and see David again. It was great having her home for a while. She is now doing a six-month internship at a Seattle hospital and gaining more and more confidence working with patients.

That brings us up to June. If you want to know what I did then—start back at the beginning of this letter. June was a good month.

It's now been six months since that last cancer tumor was diagnosed. I'm still on the daily chemotherapy pump . . . and life goes on . . . quite smoothly. Test results show that the radiation and chemotherapy have once again produced the desired results. My cancer blood levels continue to drop. Thank you, God, for the miracles in my life . . . including health, family, friends, and my FAITH.

Thank you for your thoughts and prayers. May God bless you as I have been blessed by you.

GRAB YOUR BAGS AND LET'S GO

This is again a look at the humorous side of life with cancer.

The suitcases were packed. The pump was attached. I grabbed my bags—that included my fanny pack and we're out the door! Passing through airport security got me personal attention—the kind you don't really want. I was delayed each time at the gate as I was asked to step out of line and be scanned by the magic wand device. Some check point guards were intensely frustrated that anyone would be so foolish as not to take off a fanny pack when proceeding through the buzzer gate. They would point to my guilty black bag as my passage through the walk through metal detector set the buzzer off. "You can't wear that!" they'd say with that official, abrupt voice of importance.

"I have to!" I'd say as I looked them in the eye. Then I'd see that their eyes were not looking at my eyes but at the offending black bag, which presented suspiciously. So I would undo the buckle and pull it far enough from my body that the IV tubing was exposed. Some of them got the message right away, others needed more explanation. It was unanimous at all check points that I would be pulled out of line and scanned. Legs apart, arms stretched out at my shoulders, which was proper procedure except for one poor, nervous guard who just looked at the tubing protruding from the bottom of my shirt and waved me on extra hurriedly, as if to whisk away any potential capacity for indecent exposure. Another one got alarmed and told me to stop pulling the bag away from my body—like maybe I was going to pull the tube out of the vein and start bleeding all over the checkpoint area. Another guard seemed really curious. Their job has to be rather monotonous anyway. He wanted to see the pump and the bag of IV fluids. Another woman guard offered me a wheelchair—I had to laugh after the frantic pace and suitcase scurrying I had effectively managed. It was difficult to explain to some of the security guards that the pump and IV was not detachable from my body. Another offered to hold the bag for me, but then realized that it wouldn't work with him on one side of the wall and me on the other!

Jan. 2001

THE NIGHT BEFORE CHRISTMAS

*This begins as a journal talking about Mimi's day, but ends giving us
a glimpse of the humor that Mimi displayed throughout her illness.*

January 2, 2001

I met with my Masterminds group at 7 A.M. at Marie Calland-
ers. There are six of us now who meet weekly at this time to affirm and
encourage one another. Today we each set forth our goals for the day,
week, and year. Caroline, ever college professor, passed out an outline
that we may choose to use personally to facilitate this end. I'll probably
use it as part of my discipline to be more disciplined. One of my New
Year's goals is *daily* journal writing. I've already done it for two days
now (what is it—three weeks, it is said, and it will become a habit—19
days to go and I should have it).

This group consists of motivational writers and speakers; it
forms a small capability for networking, but mostly I'd say we are
refining the art of friendship and caring about improving ourselves
and expanding that to helping others, each in our unique way. I've
been involved for about six months and am still trying to figure out
what I'm doing there. The first week I realized that it has been years
since I was up, dressed, out of the house, and functional at 7 A.M. Not
all realizations are earth-shattering by everyone's standards, but the
friends in this group understood my sense of accomplishment. I love
people who understand.

This truly is a group of compassionate women. We all have
goals of great achievements, yet we admit weekly (but not weakly—
we're honest!) to not accomplishing all our goals. One of my realizations during the six months has been that my list of goals is probably
unrealistic in view of my physical stamina at this time. After several
weeks of setting high level goals and not accomplishing very many,
I discovered that I was the main cause of most of my frustration, and
that I was setting myself up for failure. I was making myself discouraged. I announced after several months that I felt it was okay to be
a turtle. Slow but steady can work for me. Everybody smiled . . . but
didn't scoff. Nobody laughed. Some pointed out that their lists contained week after week the same unaccomplished goals . . . only eventually did those goals get accomplished. Eventually is ok so long as we

keep heading in the right direction. Satisfaction in small things can be preferable to great accomplishment with no time to assimilate. I just might be the lead turtle. Perhaps I've taught some others that it's all right to withdraw into your shell, sit on rocks much of the day, and swim when you get too hot or you want a little exercise. It's not a bad life . . . but you do have to learn to be content with the pace.

By 10:30 I was at my second appointment of the day. My goodness, how efficient! I saw Sue Helper. She wasn't rushed. She must have had time to relax over the holiday. We both appreciated having our adult children at home for the holidays. I told her about my shoulder pain, back spasms, and sciatica, and I was relieved by her broader approach to the problem. The shoulder pain appeared to her to be a likely scapular tendonitis, likely to be helped by physical therapy. I find that so much more appealing than doing back and bone scans to rule out bone metastases. I'll do both physical therapy and bone scans, but the physical therapy will feel good—in the meantime, I'll stop stewing about the bone scans. My CEA is rising so I know the scans are important. I'm just not in a hurry for them. I'm a turtle and that's ok.

Sue also entertained my theory that the back spasms and sciatica in early December that still persist to a lesser degree, may have been initiated by a combination of events. Chemo on Wednesday of that week, a Leukine (my first ever) shot on Thursday, the recent initiation of low dose Zoloft with possible sides of muscle tremors, nausea and diarrhea, and insomnia—all of which I seem to have had at once. My back went berserk—and my brain being so closely related got nervous too! Sue understood and was sympathetic. She also understands the intricacies of my back since spinal surgery and felt that it is likely that this contributed also to the spasms. She says to continue taking Baclofen if it helps. When I told Sue that despite the bone pain, I thought the switch to Neupogen shots was making me more energetic, she said that was certainly possible. Low white counts can make people tired. I have basically had white counts ranging from 2.000 to 5,000 for the past year and a half. Perhaps it is more the fatigue and lethargy of low counts and not so much depression that has gotten me down lately. That was an encouraging thought. .

To backtrack just a bit, this is the story with my back spasms. In early December (Dec. 8) part of my body (my back) wanted to lay down in a fetal position to stretch out my lower back vertebra; part of my body (my leg) needed to be straight to stop that sciatica from dancin.' Just what do you do when part of your body needs to be straight and the other part needs to be crooked??? Talk about a mental dilemma! My

poor brain got plain worn out just thinking about that—it was like trying to separate two bickering, little children joined at the hip.

Speaking of hip . . . here's another little amusing thing I was
contemplating once I got put on Vicodin and Baclofen. That stuff alters
your thinking, for sure. Since I was stuck in bed, afraid that if I moved
the leg and back those spasms might start again, I just slept on and
off . . . and did some silly thinking in between. I was thinking that I
needed to get the Christmas tree put up . . . sort of hard from a bed
position. So I was making up poetry in my head instead. T'was the
night before Christmas . . . and visions of sugarplums danced through
their heads. Only my poem was contorted a bit by my circumstances:

> . . . And visions of Leukine shots danced through her head
> And Mimi in her 'kerchief, and Tony in his cap
> Had just settled their brains for a long winter's nap.
> When in Mimi's back there arose such a clatter,
> She tried to spring from the bed to see what was the matter,
> More rapid than eagles the spasms they came.
> As she whistled and shouted and called them by name!
> (names not to be repeated)
> When what to her wondering mind did occur but a thought.

NOTE: *Here the rhyming words stopped and free form thinking took over.*

> Scientific theory started to form as I put together bits
> and pieces
> of what I knew.
> I had heard the Leukine can produce bone pain because the
> marrow has to work hard.
> I know hip and leg bones have some of the best marrow.
> My hip didn't hurt very much, but my back was killing me.
> Oh my goodness, Do you know where your hipbone is, Mimi?
> Hmm . . . the thigh bone is connected to the hip bone
> the hip bone is connected to the back bone.
> That's for most people, but not for ME!!!
> I am FEARFULLY and wonderfully made—my hipbone IS in
> my backbone!
> I have seven spinal fusions taken from my hip,
> Imagine those poor nonworking fusion places
> being lazy with spinal rods supporting them

for the past eight years, just sitting there . . .
Until they got hit with a Leukine shot . . .
They must have been so confused—
they probably forgot they were backbones now
and they started to kick out that bone marrow like
dutiful hip.
TALK ABOUT BEING WAKENED
FROM A LONG WINTER'S NAP???
Those silly bones have been snoozin' in there
for eight years . . .
and then they got called up for duty unexpectedly
in the middle of the night
Unprepared were they.
Unprepared was I.

Sept. 1997

HANDS FULL OF ENCOURAGEMENT

This story gives us all a picture of what it is like to wake up from surgery.
Mimi has done a wonderful job here in giving us an insider's perspective.

I remember coming out of the cloud of anesthesia and searching through my brain for a clue. Where was I? It hurt to breathe and I
wanted to drift back to the coma state of anesthesia, but the pain was
too powerful. I waited for the wave to pass, but it never did. The persistent pain in my left side dragged me back into reality. I wanted to
open my eyes, but I was afraid of what I might see. I have never liked
to look at hospital rooms. They make me feel weak and sick, but I knew
now I was in one of them, and I did feel weak. I could not will my eyes
to open. I did feel sick.

My left side kept hurting as I waited for this wave of pain to
pass, but the pain stayed. I had had enough surgeries in the past two
years to have learned that tensing up does nothing to relieve the pain.
Pain, I had learned, was best left to run its course while your mind did
whatever it could to distract itself. I heard the voices of my family in
the room and they were talking loud trying to wake me up, laughing
about the dinner they just had and telling me how much I missed out
on. They were familiar and sounded light-hearted and happy—all six
of them!

Momentarily, I forgot the pain as I tried to concentrate on their
words. They didn't say anything about my surgery, but I knew them all
well enough to know they wouldn't be making light-hearted conversation about their Chinese dinner if my procedure had not gone well.
I knew the surgeon's report to them must have been good, the cancer was gone from my adrenal gland and no further spread had been
found. I rested in that knowledge and drifted back under the influence
of post-anesthesia morphine relief.

Anesthesia cannot eliminate pain for very long, however, and I
woke up again to the voices of the people I loved. I hurt; my eyes still
wouldn't open. I wanted to tell my husband, cousin, and kids that I was
all right, but I couldn't figure out how to form the words. I grimaced
and adjusted my body to compensate for the pain. Then I collapsed
into the bed defeated. I was so tired of battling this disease. In the past
two years I had been in the hospital at least ten times for medical pro-

cedures related to metastatic cancer. Emerging from surgery is always a hard time of acceptance. No comfort, no self-uttered words, no eyes that open to see the light, but I felt the love. . . .

1997

CHRISTMAS LOVE

This story of Christmas demonstrates the importance of family to Mimi.

One Christmas I will never forget was three years ago. In 1994 December came while my Thanksgiving turkey tablecloth was still on the table. I didn't care, for I did not fully comprehend the passage of days. Simply getting up and dressed and walking to the kitchen was challenge enough for me. There was always someone else in the house and connecting with them in conversation took all my concentration. Two different people seemed to be living inside my head, and I was trying hard to make them one again.

Surgery two days before Thanksgiving had removed a large tumor from the frontal lobes of my brain. It still hurt to move my eyes. My speech got easily slurred, and words and thoughts dropped from my memory before I could say them. My brain would take off and race like a wild horse sometimes, and I was struggling to tame it. When I was tired or over stimulated, it sounded as if helicopter rotor blades were circling inside my skull. Other times, my mind was sluggish and slow, operating with an echo effect, and I could not cancel out the echo. I was trying hard to sort out the confusion of the world in which I lived at the moment and coping with undesirable side effects of the anti-seizure medication I needed to take while my brain was healing.

My husband's gentle patience was tangible as he attempted to guard my recovery, yet leave me room to rediscover and recreate myself. Our four grown children became models of how to do things as I watched them carefully and remembered familiar patterns of behavior. All this learning made me tired and I had to sleep a lot—sometimes for short times in the chair, often for long times in my bed. I understood how it must feel to be very old.

I also understood how it feels to be very young. I felt the tenderness and the nurturing, the hugs, and the handholding reserved in our society for the child and for those in love. A special memory is one of resting in my bed when one of my teenagers came into the cold room and snuggled under the covers with me to get warm. Moments later a second child, seeking the whereabouts of his sibling, discovered us both under the covers, lifted the blankets, and joined us in the king-size bed. The laughter brought the other two big kids into the room.

Amused by the sight, they, of course, hopped in too. Shortly afterward, my husband drifted in and said in his gruff Papa Bear voice, "Who's been sleeping in my bed?" Then he plopped down on top of three kids, who dramatically feigned suffocation, then laughed hysterically. I thought back to those days in the Midwest not so long ago when babies crawled in bed with us on stormy nights. These grown babies were conquering fear; they were learning how to handle the storms of life. They were laughing and loving instead of withdrawing. They were unleashing my emotional response, the openness, the delight, and the uninhibited responses of a child's mind. I was feeling very much loved and "in love" again.

Removal of the tumor from the area of my brain controlling personality had allowed emotions too long suppressed to emerge. Excitement and enthusiasm were returning to my life after a hiatus of at least several years. I could feel them marching back into my brain like soldiers returning to guard duty after a period of slumber. It was fun to allow these characters to dance once again through my head. They were happy, exuberant emotions like the ones I had often felt when I was younger. God emerged from within my soul and took a paramount position in my mind. I experienced ecstatic moments of His presence.

I couldn't leave the house to Christmas shop that year, and thus I experienced more fully the true meaning of Christmas. Christmas arrived in the form of a friend who came and folded up my harvest colored Thanksgiving tablecloth and replaced it with a lovely gift of red and green table covers. Christmas approached in the figures of friends who brought gifts of silken scarves and warm winter hats to keep my bald head happy. Christmas came as the Parcel Postman delivered a fluffy quilt crafted by good friends from out of town. Christmas arrived in the cookie tins, cards, wishes, and prayers of many. Christmas was there as friends arranged their schedules and came to sit with me, giving my family members the necessary time to tend to their jobs, schoolwork, and high school basketball practice. Friends sat and read or prayed by my side while I slept. They listened compassionately when my fast paced thoughts ran quicker than my ability to say them. They brought poinsettias and pretty Christmas decorations, sat and had tea and cookies with me, and left the warmth of their love to savor.

Christmas came as our two out of town college kids drifted into the driveway. Christmas came closer as they tied a big, fat Christmas tree to the top of their compact car and laughed merrily all the way home. Christmas snuck in as our kids secretly shopped, wrapped gifts, and placed them under the tree for one another. Christmas was growing in our hearts.

By Christmas Eve my heart was ready to explode. Scarcely could it hold the joy contained therein. I was overcome by so much kindness. I watched in awe as my husband and children laughed and goofed around as if to entertain me. It was a puzzling and humbling experience to be so much an observer of the family whose lives I had been instrumental in creating. I tried to feel guilty that my health was a cause for concern to the people I loved, but my family would not accept that. I had seen our children grow into adulthood right before my eyes as they emerged the caring and wonderful young people God created them to be. They made my desire to live so strong that dying was not an alternative I could choose. The fabric of our family tapestry was woven tighter, and I wanted my contribution, my flimsy threads, to remain a vital part of it. I asked God to help me.

Christmas is an easy time to ask for things. Secular society can go to Santa Claus. Christians can go to the manger to witness the depths of what God will give. God had given me everything I could have wanted. He had given me a life that I could never again take for granted. He had created in me the ability to be a survivor. Sitting there that Christmas Eve, I thought about my recent challenges and the work of God manifested in my life. Just two years earlier, through the hands of a gifted surgeon, He had corrected my spinal deformity in a ten-hour operation. With family support, my back was healing perfectly. Then just six months prior to this Christmas Eve, all six of us family members had huddled together again around my hospital bed to hear the word "Cancer" uttered in reference to my colon and liver. Further surgery and months of chemotherapy had followed, and I was still feeling the side effects. Fine doctors, a supportive family, understanding friends, and strong faith were carrying us all through this trial. Now just one month before this night, I had undergone five hours of complex brain surgery, and here I was once again on the mend.

I knew I could survive, but I worried about my husband and the burdens he must bear at work and at home keeping up family morale. I fretted about my children, all young adults. I could no longer protect them from the inevitable realities of a world that is sometimes difficult to comprehend. In my quiet times, though, I could see that God protected them, as He always had. As we gathered around the Christmas tree that Christmas Eve and shared gifts and celebrated the birth of Jesus, we could feel the Love of God. We had experienced the Hope He promised. To those who seek Him, we understood the Peace He gave.

We had these gifts of Love and Hope and Peace. As Christmas Day drifted into the day after, these gifts remained with us to be opened and discovered, uncovered, and shared. These are the gifts I wish all of you this Christmas. May you be surrounded by those you Love. * May you find the Peace the Son of God brought and left with us.** May you cling to His promise of Hope to a world gone astray.*** Go to the manger. You will find all these gifts. A very Merry Christmas to you all.

> * For God so loved the world that He gave His one and only Son.
> John 3:16

> **Peace I leave with you; My peace I give you.
> John 14:27

> ***And we rejoice in the hope of the glory of God. Not only so, but we also rejoice in our sufferings, because we know that suffering produces perseverance; perseverance, character; and character, hope. And hope does not disappoint us, because God has poured out His love into our hearts by the Holy Spirit, whom He has given us.
> Romans 5:2-5

June 2001

ANGELS

*The beginning of this letter gives us a glimpse of Mimi's
unorganized side. When Tony was going through
Mimi's stuff, he found these Christmas letters.*

June 2, 2001

Dear Aunt Mimi and Uncle Joe,

Oh my, oh, my . . . how does the time go by so fast????

I still have Christmas cards I haven't sent . . . from 1999!!! I sent you one , it's the one with the family picture. I never got any cards out in 2000 . . . because I was going to send the rest of the 1999 cards to the people that never got them in 1999. Get it!

I had a nice Get Well card for Uncle Joe in January. It has a droopy dog on the front and a funny saying on the inside. I was going to mail that back in January when he was facing surgery and all the other unpleasant accompaniments to colon cancer. I'm sorry you have to go through all that, Uncle Joe . . . but just hang in there!!! I've been dealing with the same beast for seven years—the surgery, chemotherapy, and radiation. I guess you could say that I am living proof that the doctors do know what works. You never seem to feel to good going through it—sick, sleepy, sedated . . . but ever smiling!!! That's the secret.

I've been keeping track of you, Uncle Joe, from the various members of my family who have seen you at family gatherings. They say you are still the same dedicated, sweet man as always . . . and that a weakened body does not dampen your hard working, stick with it, dedicated attitude. I know it has taken a great deal of effort and patience to rehabilitate and face the demon of cancer—but you and I know that God can help us through these trials. You've been in my constant prayers. We all love you so much.

I thought it would be nice to send you a Valentine. I might have actually accomplished that because I know I bought a package of cute ones at the card store . . . and they sat on my kitchen table for about two weeks, and whenever I had a chance I addressed a couple and mailed them. The problem is, I had no sense of order . . . and I don't know who got them and who didn't. So if you got one, Congratulations! If not—Belated Happy Valentine's.

I didn't even buy St. Patrick's Day cards. I knew better, **but I did have St. Patrick's stickers,** and I thought I'd just attach them to the Valentine's cards I didn't send . . . but by then the Valentine's cards were lost someplace because we had had house guests, Rita (Jennings) Newton from Milwaukee stopped by with her husband on their way to visit their son who now goes to school out here in California. It was great to see Rita after nearly 25 years. We were both majoring in physical therapy at Marquette—she was three or four years behind me! You never know when family members will show up on your doorstep! Anyway, when Rita and Mike came, I cleaned up the kitchen table and put the Valentine and St. Patrick's stickers away in some safe storage place . . . and they haven't been discovered yet.

When Easter came, I was so ashamed that I've been delinquent in the corresponding department that **I went out and bought a really nice card with flowers on the front,** and as you see I managed to update it and that's the one you have just received. Isn't it nice??????

Aunt Mimi, I was so sad to hear about you having a small stroke last month. Especially, when I heard that you'd had a stroke, I felt bad because I know how much you hate all those tests and needles and any other procedures. Those actually can make you feel sicker than the stroke itself, huh?? I am wired that same way as you—I feel sick when I see the needles coming at me. I'm getting real used to it though—and any more I just act like I'm donating my body to science, and I let the doctors do their stuff while my mind goes skipping off to someplace fun like the Twin Lakes Beach at Family Reunion Time in June.

By the way I have recently received your lovely invitation to yet another fun party at the lake, but once again I won't be able to make it. I've just had a few weeks off chemotherapy . . . and now I'm back on it again, and I have to be cautious about getting overtired or exposed to too many germs. I know none of the people coming to your party have germs, but you just can't trust the crowds in the airport and on the planes.

Despite my recent rounds of radiation and chemotherapy, I have had some times when I was feeling very well and Tony and I have been able to do some traveling recently. In February, he and I went to a meeting in Las Vegas. David was able to drive from San Diego (three hours) and met us there. Julie Davy came to our hotel and we all had a fun lunch.

In April we went to a medical meeting in San Diego for several days. We were able to spend the weekend with David and his girlfriend Robin (good for each other, neither ready for wedding bells!) and we had dinner with my cousin Gail Gardner (Cass and Hugh's daughter) while we were there. That was a really fun weekend. David had just returned from two weeks in Japan where he presented a lecture on the work he and his team are currently doing at Sun Microsystems. He toured Tokyo, which is a modern Japanese City and also went to Kyoto, which is a more traditional, ancient city. He visited museums, toured the city, visited the shrines, enjoyed a performance at the Cherry Blossom festival, spent a day with our Japanese friends who lived next door to us in St. Louis and moved back to Tokyo in 1990, and he was not afraid to eat raw fish. It was fun to hear about his trip.

Liz was home for spring break. When Liz left to go back to school, Katie was able to be free on Easter weekend so she came home. David was in Japan, Liz was back in Tacoma, and Chris was in Wisconsin on call at her Lancaster hospital . . . but Katie sometimes thinks it's fun to be an only child for a weekend. UCLA, where she works, is two hours south of Bakersfield so she comes home sometimes when she has two days off. She is very busy in her pediatrics residency and is happy that her first year is almost over. She has two more years to go, and then she'll be out in practice as a pediatrician.

I was able to jump on a shuttle flight to Las Vegas in late April—cheap, two hours by air—and I spent three days with five of my girlfriends from St. Louis. We laughter a lot and lost a little cash but had a great time. This is the group I get together with almost every year. I spent my last night in Las Vegas with Julie Davy. She is a delightful hostess, and I got to hear all about her new flame, Josh.

On the last weekend in April, I walked in the Relay for Life to raise funds for the American Cancer Society. Uncle Joe, I was walking with you on my mind. I do hope that your cancer is under control. I understand that you have been an admirable patient, and that you are continuing to get stronger. Keep it up—the world needs your inspiration!!!

Our last trip was up to Tacoma for Liz's graduation. The big day was also Mother's Day. Having Tony, David, and Katie present for the college graduation of our baby made it a really special day for all of us. It's hard to get all six of us together—but five out of six is not bad. Tony and I stayed in Washington for an extra week after graduation and took Liz on a road trip of the Olympic Peninsula. For four days we traveled and hiked through the tall sequoia trees, the rain forest, and the beautiful beaches with huge tree trunks washed up on the beaches, bleached by years in the sun and looking like huge old white dinosaur skeletons on the beach. It's gorgeous country up there.

Liz will remain in Tacoma and Seattle for the next six months because she has to complete six months of school-supervised internships before she can be board certified in occupational therapy. Then she is not sure whether she'll stay in Washington, come back to California, or go elsewhere. Much depends on the job market.

Thank you for thinking of Liz on her Graduation Day. She got beautiful cards from you and Joe and Gina . . . and, of course, the monetary bonuses are much appreciated . . . especially prior to the beginning of a paying job!

I was sorry to hear of Uncle Tom's death upon our return from Tacoma. I knew that he had been very sick. My mom, Sue, and the boys keep me updated. I had received a letter from Donna after her birthday and she had asked for prayers for her father as his health was failing. The death of those we love is always so sad. I know it has been hard on the family with Aunt Virginia's accident and all the related problems before her death and with Uncle Tom's failing health resulting in hospitalization. I thank God for the hope we can all have that we will one day all be united with Him . . . We are all people of faith and know this is true, but it is still so difficult to say good-bye to the ones we love. Those brothers of yours, Aunt Mimi, were really special guys . . . they taught us all so much . . . about life . . . with laughter . . . and with love . . . with family and with Faith. We still see them shine through you. Keep smiling, even through the tears, because I know the boys are singing together again. I often picture my dad just smiling at me. I still see his blue eyes and his chubby cheeks, and I feel his perseverance and his patience. I know he is happy in Heaven. He and Uncle Bob and Uncle Tom always thought this life was a fine place too. They were perfect models of gentle men . . . and their lessons continue to come across to us . . . they'll always have loving influence upon us.

My love and prayers unite me with you and Uncle Joe. May you both continue to experience improved health in your comfortable new condominium . . . and some awesome sunsets at the lake this summer. I'll be thinking of you on the twenty-third of June!!! Please give my love to all. We truly have been blessed with a wonderful loving family.

God Bless us, Everyone.

Late 2001

We again get to see Mimi's disorganized side.

Oh my, oh my, oh my . . . my intentions were good,
But . . .

I started the enclosed epistle just after my birthday last June. I thought that since I had never gotten around to mailing Christmas cards last year that it might be nice to send an update six months **after** Christmas. That just happens to be my birthday—June 25 . . . so I wrote a little birthday memory with a combined thank you to the people who made my birthday so special.

I thought it was just going to be a short note, but it turned into seven pages! Then I thought seven pages sounded a little wordy and probably a bit pompous, so I thought that I would just leave it in my computer as a personal journal entry. I thought I would edit parts for individual's letters. I tried that . . . and ended up losing some of the good stuff. I don't have a lot of patience or expertise in thinking like a computer—so I climb into bed and take a nap whenever I have the feeling that the computer is being unfriendly. I always hope that I will wake up knowing everything there is to know about working a computer. It hasn't happened yet . . .

Then a couple weeks ago, I wanted to send a letter to a friend (Bob McNulty) who was playfully griping that I never answered his birthday phone call . . . and it was three months after our mutual birthday already! I told Bob that I was sorry to be so slow, but I would write him a letter soon; I promised. Well, the days went by and I never wrote him that letter. Then I thought—Ha! Ha! I know what I will do. I'll print up my birthday journal thoughts—where it just so happened that I mentioned his phone call—and I will send him all seven pages!!!! He may think I am slow about responding, but he'll know at least I'm thorough . . .

So I mailed my letter to Bob. I thought I better mail one to my sister and my mom too . . . because they would be talking to Bob . . . and might wonder why he got a letter and they didn't.

Well, they called me all excited . They liked the letter. It didn't matter that it was four months late. So I just went and made copies . . . and that's the same letter you're getting because I am too lazy to write anymore letters . . .

I will, however, update you as to what has happened since June . . .

In July I had a ten-day break from the 24-hour-a-day chemotherapy pump, and I was able to obtain tickets to fly back to Wisconsin to visit Christine. She was still recovering from mono and was struggling with the back to work routine. I went back to play mom and friend. Neither of us had what you would call an excess of energy, but we thoroughly enjoyed just spending the week together. Friends stopped in, and we worked together on redoing all her yellowed baby albums . . . and turned them into beautiful, creative memory pages. One night while we were working together with a group of her friends, one of the young mothers in the group asked me, "What would I change if I could do anything over again?"

I thought for a while and answered, "Nothing. Because, you see, I am looking at these photos of a baby I had thirty years ago (Happy Birthday, Christine) . . . and now I have just fast-forwarded ahead 30 years into my future. The baby is grown, a respectable adult, and she is happy. You can't ask for much more than that . . ." It was a rather revealing insight. It's a small glimpse of what God knows. He can hold us as an infant . . . and know exactly where we will be 30 . . . and 60 and 100-plus years into the future. Cool, huh?

August was hot here. I was either wading in the swimming pool (couldn't get my IV needle wet) or in the air-conditioning. Heat does not mix well with chemotherapy. I continued with a few more days of playing teacher with my little 6-year-old triplet friends, and I tried hard to get back into writing some of my personal journal experiences. My friend Marcia broke her hip, and I was able to help her out some, with hospital and rehab spirit-lifting visits. When she got home, I could help her out with meals a little bit. Marcia is one of the women in our church. She and I have done some writing and editing together. She's just the type of uplifting fun person I need. Even though I have reduced activity, I was a step more efficient in simple maneuvers than Marcia at that time.

September was an exciting month. Tony received his Fellowship Award in the American College of Radiology. The presentation was in San Francisco and Katie, David, and Liz were able to meet us there. (Christine couldn't get anymore time off work because the mono had made her associates feel "overburdened.") We all met on Sunday, celebrated being together; had a great time on Monday touring the Museum of Modern Art . . . and looked forward to the ceremony the next night (Tuesday).

Tuesday morning we were awaken to the sad and distressing news of the terrorist attack on the Pentagon and the Trade Center. We gathered in front of the TV and watched the events of the day unfold—in sorrow, grief, and shock. It was the worst TV "show" we have ever watched. We only wished it was only a show . . .

The Fellowship ceremony went on as planned that evening, but it was converted into a much more subdued and patriotic event. Two of the honorary members were from Europe. The physician from Spain was unable to deliver his prepared speech but simply said, "A terrible crime has happened in your country today. My speech would not be right in light of this event. I am from a country that has suffered under oppression. I can only express to you I'm sorry." It was one of the most sincere, short, noble speeches I've heard. The other speaker was a 70-year-old doctor from Poland who had brought modern cancer therapy back to Poland during World War II. He had been an outspoken anti-communist, and he tried to get funding for his research. He spoke very sensitively about the trials and difficulty of trying to help people survive in a country at war. Both these men gave a sense of hope and perspective to the new world situation we were facing on this September 11, 2001. Message: The human heart and our God allow us to Hope . . . and In God we MUST trust.

My mom was supposed to have flown out here to California on Sept. 11, 2001. Fortunately, she had not yet boarded the plane or she would have been diverted to Canada. She would have driven the Canadian authorities nuts! She bravely rescheduled her departure for Sunday of that same week—no terrorists were going to keep her from seeing her kids in California and Bud and Lynn's two new grandbabies (her great-grandchildren in Riverside, CA). Well, O'Hare airport had the nerve to cancel her flight, and she now is rescheduled for Thanksgiving week out here in California. It was sad that she was unable to come in September, but the fact that planes were grounded meant that Liz could not fly back to Tacoma either. Katie and David both had the weekend off . . . so Liz, Katie, David, and I all went to Riverside for the mini-family reunion that was to have been in honor of my mom. We saw Joe and Diana's new house and we held those new babies . . . and MJ got a photo album to look at . . . until she can get out her and see for herself in November.

Now it's almost the end of October. I am happy that the weather has turned cooler. I have more energy. I'm still on the chemotherapy pump 24 hours a day for three weeks, then I have a week or two off to recover. I've been maintaining this therapy for seven months . . . and I've aged about seven years worth. My cancer has not been totally killed yet, but then, neither have I!!! That's a positive. This is a mean disease, but I'm still keeping up with the treatment, and my condition has remained stable for the past five months. My doctors seem encouraged. So am I . . . most of the time.

I wish I had more time and energy to keep up with friends like you, but I've been hanging out with the Bible on tape during my lazy days, sponsoring a new candidate for the RCIA process in the Catholic Church, and being an aide in the Elementary Religious Education first grade classroom where my three little triplets buddies are learning about God. I'm not bored . . . and sometimes life is hard, but God is Good.

Sept. 1998

LABOR DAY 1998

Dear Friends,

Well, today marked the official end of summer, and I am sitting here doing some reflecting so I thought I'd write it down. Then I will mail it to my friends . . . and they will all understand why I have not corresponded with many people this summer.

It was quite an eventful summer—

In mid-May, after Liz got out of school, she came home to Bakersfield for three weeks so she could have ankle surgery on an old basketball injury. The surgery went well, though for the rest of the summer she continued to have fluid accumulating in the joint with lots of pain. (I'm sure it had nothing to do with the fact that she returned to a busy summer job of coaching 5- to 14-year-olds for six hours a day at Sports Camps throughout the Seattle/Tacoma area—not exactly a sedentary job!) At this age, kids just feel like they can't take time out of living to heal properly. Personal experience is the best teacher. I guess they must learn these lessons for themselves, the hard way.

Liz did remain in Bakersfield for a two-week recovery period and was able to go with the family to my nephew's wedding in Riverside, California (about three hours from Bakersfield). Although Liz, Katie, David, and I were able to be there, Tony and Christine were not. Christine had her farewell to residency party at the hospital that same evening, and Tony was home recovering from angioplasty that had been performed four days earlier on a blocked heart vessel. Like we needed a few more health insurance claims in this family!!!! (Unlike Liz, who was impatient and rarin' to go full speed ahead after surgery, Tony was quite content to "relax" and "not do any physical things like exercise for fear it will strain his heart.) Fortunately, his doctor is aware of his aversion to exercise so he placed him in cardiac rehab so he gets a workout at least twice a week. I am thankful for that though Tony is not necessarily happy with the fact that he has to go in at 6:30 A.M. before work.

Most of my family had flown out from Chicago for my nephew's wedding so I was excited to be there. Katie and David both got the weekend off from school and joined their cousins and had a ball! I loved seeing and being with everyone and was thankful that Christine was home to watch after her dad. I stayed in Riverside for the Irish wedding celebration for three days. Then I brought some of the relatives back here to Bakersfield and enjoyed a couple days with them.

In late June Tony did take time off work, and he and I drove up to Carmel and Monterey Bay (close to where we all went on our Playgroup excursion four years ago) where we celebrated my birthday. By the way, thank you all for remembering my birthday. Your calls and cards really meant a lot to me. This year was a rather reflective birthday as it also marked my fourth year as a cancer survivor—I've had four years of accumulated prayers . . . and God continues to bless me so much with a supportive family and wonderful, very special friends (as Kay says—friends are flowers that never fade). Thanks.

I knew I was in for a tough summer course of chemotherapy after my June vacations—and my oncologist did not disappoint me!!! My dose was raised (that was his contribution). I switched to automatic pilot mode (that was my contribution—it's where judgment bypasses the brain) and scheduled my frustrated self for extra weeks of chemo at the high dose. I was so frustrated by a full year of non-stop chemo with a steady, though slow, rise in my CEA (Cancer antigen indicator in my blood) that I decided to take matters into my own hands and try to "Whip this bast—d disease" by not taking the prescribed breaks from chemo . . .

Those extra weeks of chemo with no recovery period special ordered by "DOCTOR" Mimi Deeths actually made me sick, but I didn't know it because I can do this auto-pilot thing pretty good (where you just fool your brain and the people around you into thinking you are fine when you are not). I was sleeping much more than usual (blamed it on the heat). My hands were turning reddish-black (blamed it on the hot Bakersfield sun). I was sweating all the time (just drank more water). My eyes were burning and would not stop tearing (wore cool blue shades)! Even my eyebrows began to fall out (so I just bought eyebrow pencils). Then the nurses caught on to what I was doing; the doctor returned from vacation—and they all thought that I should let them be in charge of ordering my treatment!!! I was ordered off chemo entirely for a month. They said I had become toxic and my body needed a recovery period. My hands were not sunburned but drug (acid) burned and the lethargy was due to my liver not being able to process all the drug fast enough, low potassium, and a depressed immune system.

It took me two or three weeks to recover, but it felt really good being off the "stuff." I took advantage of the time-off period and spent extra time with Christine as she prepared to move back to Wisconsin.

After she moved on August 4, I drove down to spend a couple days with my brother and his family in Riverside, spent a long afternoon with David in San Diego, and stayed overnight with Katie who had just moved into a house with two other med students in Long Beach. I felt good and had a wonderful time . . . forgetting about the chemo bad days, Tony's heart problems, and Christine's moving from Bakersfield. It was sort of like the two-day "fantasy land" Playgroup adventures we do—just fun where we can forget we are the ages we are. I hung out with the kids' younger crowd for a few days. I miss that on a regular basis so it was great fun . . . but I must say I was happy to return to my empty nest at the end of exhaustion so I could sleep, and I did for about three days!!!

Then it was back to the old chemotherapy routine the last week in August, and I remain on it now. I'll do six weeks in a row then have two weeks off to recover. So far I am in my second week and am tolerating the high dose quite well. I'm letting my oncologist be in charge, though both he and my psychologist gave me some credit for "wanting to take control of my disease" and not feeling like a victim. These kinds of professionals are very good at dealing with wacky people and making them feel OK about their feelings. I just figured I would test them!!! However, they don't want me to do that again. I promised I would not. I love these guys; they are so patient—and just cool about the whole thing. I also am pretty happy about my little experiment—after one year of monthly rises in my CEA level, my going toxic actually dropped the little sucker down by one point. It may not even be of any statistical significance (we'll know in a couple weeks if there is a downward pattern), but for the moment I feel that I may have accomplished something. Cancer is a weird disease—so much of it has become understood scientifically, but so much is still individual and trial and error. I trialed and errored. I still try to follow God's guidance. As you know He sometimes speaks very quietly, and we don't know for sure what He is trying to tell us, but I never heard Him shout out to me that I was getting toxic and should have a chemo rest . . . so I think he was passively approving and protecting me from danger while I did my Chemo-press in July. I love God, and I know He loves me. I feel safe. He protects me from minor infractions of the chemo rules . . . and other silly things that I do. He's given us free will, sometimes I think He wants to see how far we will go with that.

One of the other awesome wonders of the summer was that I became involved in a woman's Bible Study group right in the neighborhood. It was a wonderful group of ladies, some of whom I knew well before the study began and others that I got to know as very special friends. We began as a disciplined group and ended up as a less disciplined group because we got to love and enjoy each other so much . . . but then, we were studying the three letters of John that are largely about Christian Love . . . and I like to think we were just putting those lessons into practice! God not only allows that, I think perhaps He likes that in a Bible Study. I wonder if He is as "amused" by our ladies straying-from-the-main-point fellowship as are husbands would be???? Do you think He just rolls His eyes back in His head in mock frustration but actually approves of our female networking???

I have gotten involved this summer with Hospice Speaker's Bureau and the local branch of the Cancer Society. I had to give my first practice speech to the group of eight who comprise the Hospice Speaker's Bureau. It was like a speech class critique. The consensus was that most of them were holding back tears, and although my delivery was less than professional, my sincerity came through so that I was very convincing. Like most of the groups I am involved in, I love the people and have fun, though speaking on sensitive and serious subjects. We have all been trying to read the book *Tuesdays with Morrie* by Mitch Albom because it works well into the hospice concept. I would highly recommend it to anyone of you who hasn't read it. It was a #1 bestseller for a while this summer. I've given a copy to my kids because I think it is a great life- reference book for them. I'm also on the planning committee for a Woman to Woman series for the Cancer Society. We will have community lectures open to the public once a month dealing with issues such as hormones, nutrition, visualization and relaxation, advances in cancer research, radiation therapy, etc. This fall my oncologist's group is opening a multi-million dollar Comprehensive Cancer Center here in Bakersfield, and I think there will be more community awareness and support.

This weekend (Labor Day) was a perfect end to summer. My mom had made a great recovery from thyroid surgery and a very good adjustment to the retirement home. Tony seems to be handling his heart condition with far less anxiety. Christine is settled in Wisconsin, seems reasonably secure, and is noticing and enjoying the benefits of the small town extended-family feeling. Katie began her third-year med school in July, and so she is now in the hospital full-time. The first weeks were tough as she called home and said, "I've never liked being in hospitals. They just make me feel sick. I hate working in the hospital everyday and night too!" I wrote her a "mom" letter told her that hospitals are useful when seen through the eyes of someone in the bed as

I have been. I was flattered when she read excerpts of my letter at the noon conference she presented on Humanity in Medicine. She's feeling better generally about her ability to survive the next five (?) years in the hospital. David will be entering his second senior year in late September, had a good time this summer, and made good money for the computer firm he's been working for two years now. Liz was home for three days between the end of her summer job and the beginning of school—after completing three years of undergraduate study, she's looking forward to beginning her 2 1/2 year occupational therapy curriculum. She just moved into a campus house with four other girls over this Labor Day weekend.

Though Christine and Elizabeth were not here for the Holiday weekend, David and Katie came up from their respective schools with friends who took over Chris and Liz's rooms so we had a great houseful of enthusiastic 20-something kids. Tony and I enjoyed the excitement of cooking for ten (I can't keep up with Mother Jones a.k.a. JoAnn), and then we were ready to send them off on their way to demanding school schedules . . . and relax in our empty nest. I've learned to like this state of being and thank God for the satisfaction that comes from watching our children grow into happy and responsible, respectful adults . . . You all know how good that feels . . .

I hope you have all enjoyed a satisfying summer . . . and fly into your new fall routines with anticipation of good things to come.

Mid-1999

TO BE 50

When Mimi's kids were little, she got involved in a playgroup.
Each week, six mothers would all drop their kids off at
someone's house (a different person each week),
so that they could be without the kids for awhile.
Well, these six mothers got to be friends, so after the kids
started going off to school, they still wanted to play.
They started by going to lunch together. Over time,
members moved away, so then they switched to
yearly trips to various exotic locations.

NOTE: NOW THAT I AM 50, I FORGET WHO I TOLD WHAT TO. THAT'S WHY I AM WRITING THE SAME LETTER TO ALL OF YOU . . . SO I KNOW YOU WILL ALL HAVE THE SAME INFORMATION. I SAVED A COPY FOR MYSELF SO I CAN HAVE THE SAME INFORMATION TOO . . . OTHERWISE I MIGHT FORGET NOT ONLY WHAT HAPPENED BUT WHOM I TOLD WHAT TO. GET IT???? HAPPY END OF SUMMER TO YOU ALL.

SEPTEMBER 1 (Where did the time go??????)

Dear Jeren, Betty, Kay, Joan, and Pat,

Do you realize that it's been **four months** since we were together in Destin, and Pat was over in Rome with Jack, her aunt and uncle, and Pope John Paul. By the way, Pat, we all need one photo of you in Rome to add to our Destin mementos. We thought of you—I hope they had mudslides over in Rome.

I know I am a bit delinquent, but I really have thought of writing this letter so often, but I usually take a nap instead . . . and just dream of you . . .

A couple weeks ago in the mail, I got a birthday book from Betty. She meant to mail it a couple months ago but just got around to it. I love Betty because she gets things done at a pace that I can deal with. I grabbed it on my way out the door on a car-repair-sit and wait day—and would you believe, I actually enjoyed my two hours in the customer lounge!!! I was uninterrupted, reading my book, *Friends of the*

Heart, and reminiscing once again about all the special times we have had together over the years. We are **truly blessed** to have such a friendship. I share some of the reflections with you in the enclosed notebook pages.

What I have been meaning to write for the past four months (see what I mean about liking Betty's schedule!) is "Thank you so much for arranging the surprise T-shirt idea." It was truly a surprise, great fun, and a delight to show-and-tell about, even to this day. Thank you for the fun, the free drinks, and dinner and dessert down on the ocean front on the last night we were there.

I may not have said how much I appreciated the condo set-up, but I really did! I needed those lazy, sleep-in mornings, and you gals were all so cool about just extending your morning coffee gabbing until well past noon. By then, I was ready to go and shop, sightsee, dine, drink, and play Balderdash well into the night. Wasn't that too much Fun????? I can't wait to see how Pat catches on. She will be impressed with how smart we are!

As you know, my fun sort of came to an abrupt halt soon after my return as I headed back for more scans and even a trip to UCLA to try to figure out why my cancer levels were rising more rapidly. By June 1, I was in the hospital for urological surgery where the doctors discovered a cancer tumor in the ureter near my left kidney. The surgeon blasted part of it out with a laser, put a catheter in the ureter to keep my kidney draining properly . . . and we are waiting for chemotherapy to destroy what remains of that tumor.

I e-mailed you all last week about the latest results of my CEA (cancer marker) levels. The chemotherapy did a job on my hair. Right now, I have a few little gray and white spriggles poking out of my scalp. Very sparse, and as Katie says, "Mom, I've seen better hair on a coconut!" I laugh when I look at myself. She's right. The wig is an improvement. I wore it for David's graduation (see how good I look in the photo—I think I look better than usual). The chemotherapy is doing a job on my cancer cells too. In May before surgery, they were at 80. In mid-June they were 57; in mid-July they were 27. In mid-August they were 9.9—that's the first time in two years they have been down in the single digits . Normal is 0 to 3 . . . so I'm getting close.

I wasn't even thinking about my birthday because my focus was getting through the surgery, handling the new chemotherapy, and getting to David's graduation on June 13, but during my birthday week, some friends had a surprise luncheon for fourteen of us at a local restaurant. It was rather overwhelming. So much birthday niceness . . .

Then the nicest thing of all happened . . . my kids all surprised me by coming into town on my real birthday. We spent the weekend together, and they presented me with the memory book, which all of you are well aware of. We laughed and cried together all weekend. The book of memories is such a treasured gift. The special thoughts behind it leave me in awe of God's goodness and grace.

My emotions have been on a roller coaster most of the last four months. The new chemotherapy is rougher than the last one. Sometimes I feel downright obnoxious as a result of nausea, fatigue, irritability, and gastro-intestinal explosions. (Now what kind of Balderdash word do you think we could make up for that definition? Descriptive, isn't it?) On the other hand, I have been able to enjoy many quality times this past four months . . . so the chemotherapy is not really as bad as I'm making it sound.

One of the problems is that this new stuff is administered with steroids (Decadron), and that makes me restless and probably plays a part in the emotional swings. Sometimes it makes me high, however . . . and that can be pretty fun. Never having been a drug user in the seventies, I feel sometimes like I am getting my chance now, but I would much rather get my jollies playing Balderdash and visiting outlet shops in matching birthday T-shirts . . . or something naturally silly.

One month after my birthday—on July 30—I had another birthday celebration. My friends from church had wanted to do something for my birthday in June, but I told them very honestly that with the discovery of the new cancer tumor, the new therapy, and David's graduation this was just not a good time. They respected my request . . . but insisted they wanted to celebrate my birthday anyway . . . and just postponed it by a month. When I told this church group that I frequently did not feel well, napped a lot, and sometimes had to blast off to the bathroom, they said that was ok. They would just come and clean up my house for me, bring all the food, and invite all the people **here** for a birthday BASH. Then I could go to my own bed to take a nap or use my own bathroom if necessary. Everything was fine—I was in good party mode with no exhaustion and no upheavals! It was nice. My house got clean that way too.

I had 30 friends here at my house for that 50th birthday celebration. It was wonderful. Since that was the fifth celebration of the year, I was really getting into this birthday business. I look upon the whole thing in a philosophical way. When I was 45 and newly diagnosed with cancer, one of my goals in life was just TO BE 50. I had reached that goal accompanied by the love and prayers of many . . . and this is what we were celebrating!!!!

I have since reflected on the loveliness of all my birthday celebrations and the thoughtfulness of friends who created them for me. Thank you for everything you did for my birthday. I think I'll keep celebrating all year!

August moved into more family celebrations as Tony and I and Liz all flew back to visit Christine in Lancaster. (Katie and David had been there last Christmas.) Her town is really quaint with old, two-story brick houses, volunteer fire department and rescue squad, two restaurants—A & W Root beer and Wagon Wheel Pizza, a candy bar wrapper factory, new car dealerships, a drug store, one grocery store, a flower shoppe, and a men's and women's clothing store, a big Pomeida store (that's like Wal-Mart), a bunch of churches, farms, small businesses, two medical clinics, and a roomy, 22 bed hospital with a large portrait of Christine hanging in the front hall along with the seven other doctors in the town! It is like stepping back in time. I think when I get old I will go back there to the nursing home—it's right across from the A &W Root Beer Restaurant and the nursing home residents can walk across the street and have breakfast in town! Such freedom. Maybe you would all like to move there too . . . so we could visit everyday. Christine truly loves it there, and I can see why. Not many people have the desire or courage to return willingly to a simpler place and time, but I found it to be a pleasant taste of nostalgia. It reminds Christine of the little lake town in Wisconsin where I would take the kids for a week in the summer. I still love that little town.

From Lancaster, Tony and Liz and Christine and I drove four hours north to Appleton, Wisconsin, and settled into the Village Country Inn there for the next four days. Our nephew and Godson, Matthew Deeths, married a girl from this lovely town on Lake Winnebago. Katie and David flew in from California and joined us there for four days of wedding festivities including a buffet dinner on the lakefront with Tony's brother and family, a rehearsal dinner for 60 people the following night, the wedding reception at a neat, old country club on that Saturday, and brunch for 100 people at the bride's parents' house on Sunday. It was a fun family time, more special memories . . .

Liz and Tony had to fly home on Sunday for work. Katie and Christine drove back to Lancaster. David and I rented a car and drove to Chicago to visit my family. I stayed with my mom at the Senior Center. She has slowed down a bit, but she is very happy in her new place. She has plenty of people to talk to, and Mass is offered right in the church at the retirement center every day so she gets up and dressed and off to Mass and coffee afterwards so she can keep abreast of everybody's comings and goings. Mass is a wonderful opportunity to display your daughter and grandson when they come to visit! We met the priest and loads of people, and my mom had a hard time controlling her pride—it is nice to see her so at home and happy where she is.

Each night while I was in Chicago, Mom and David and I would go to a different relative or siblings house for dinner and any one else who wanted to see us would come over too . . . so I think we visited with well over 50 family members in the three days we were there. It was such fun to see everyone; so many of our kids have just graduated recently and begun new jobs—it was fun to listen to this new generation of working people. Aren't our young people neat????? I love their freshness, their enthusiasm, and their style.

Ten days after I had flown back to the Midwest, I turned around and flew back to California. Within 18 hours of my return home, I was back to reality . . . in the oncology chair again. After such a nice vacation and time off, the chemo knocked me on my butt for a couple weeks. I had four doses between August 13 and August 31. I was not very friendly. I think I was having an attitude problem. I slept a lot and took a bunch of antinausea medication. The initial effect has worn off finally, and I'm getting to feeling better. Now . . . just thinking about all that has happened in the past four months makes me smile. I'm off chemotherapy next week so I can build up my immune system for a repeat urological surgery on June 14 (I'll be in the hospital 24–48 hours), but I'm anticipating resting and feeling good for the next ten days . . . until the surgery. Then I'll get obnoxious again. However . . . thinking about YOU, and all that my friends and family do for me, has renewed my spirit and restored my perspective. I LOVE BEING 50!!!!

Thank you for making me laugh. Thank you for being such neat friends!!!!!!!

P.S. I have had so much fun with my Birthday memory book that I thought I would start one for each of you. I've sent you the first pages—all you have to do is get yourself a three-ring binder and some more of these plastic cover sheets at any office store (Office Depot, etc. is cheaper than craft store) . . . and keep adding to it. It is fun for letters, photos, birthday cards, etc. Happy Autumn!!!

Dec. 1996

This was after another trip with her Playgroup friends.

December 1, 1996

Dear Joan,

That date above just blows my mind. I can't believe it's been six weeks since we were all at your home in Virginia. I had intended to write you right away and thank you for all of your planning and for such a wonderful time, but . . . you know how that goes. First I was going to get the photos developed and send them along with the thank-you note . . . and they didn't get out of the camera as a finished roll for three weeks. Then it was getting near Thanksgiving, so I found a cute Thanksgiving card to send . . . but Gramma and Grampa were coming up for Thanksgiving and David and Liz were coming home . . . and heavy-duty house cleaning took precedence. So here it is getting on toward Christmas, and I've decided that before Santa comes I will mail both the photos AND the Thanksgiving card!!!

Anyway, I thought the card was very appropriate with the fall leaves and the little bears. It reminded me of the East Coast leaves and our Playgroup warm, fuzzy friendship. I just value that time together. It is so incredible to me that we all met so long ago and have kept up the relationship, especially with you and me moving to opposite coasts. It feels good to think that even though you and I live as far apart almost as any users could live, we have each visited one another's houses . . . and brought those land-locked St. Louisans with us!!!!

Maybe I'm just getting old (heaven's no—not if we still have periods!!!) or maybe just more philosophical, but it is so special to look back and see where we all came from. We didn't know what we were doing 25 years ago . . . and with those babies, etc. But we shared some sanity times back then, socialized our toddlers a bit . . . and everyone of them has grown up to be a good kid. Our husbands have all remained faithful, and we've come to realize with introspective sharing with the "girls" that all men are created equal. Our husbands' quirks are normal. They are great guys. We've all relied on each other and trusted God . . . and that's the secret, I'm convinced.

In the last couple years, we've all had to deal with problems we hadn't anticipated—yours and Betty's struggles with beloved parents and Alzheimer's and related stress on the families you grew up with, who have changed course in their maturing processes—you, Brian and John Schlautman, and myself with those kinds of physical problems that don't disappear—financial woes, job changes, kids leaving home, etc. It can be a trying time—knowing how much friends care can help to lessen the struggle. I for one have had concrete proof of how much you guys care. It really means so much.

It was wonderful to see Brian and John. Brian is absolutely darling . . . and I still see so much of the little, tennis, nursery boy that Elizabeth loved in that face. His smile and his spirit have not changed. He's a survivor . . . and you'd never know by looking at him that he's ever had a battle. He just makes me proud, President of Student Council and all!! Also, tell him I am incredibly impressed at how he cleaned that room!!! It shows that the boy's been civilized. You can feel proud, Mom. I hope that all goes well with his cardiology follow-ups. He looks wonderful!

It was such fun to see your house. It's beautiful, and it was fun to see how you decorated. By the way, I found a minestrone soup mix similar to the one you had the night we arrived . . . and it was fun to fix it for the family here and remember that wonderful family feeling at your house again. Every part of the trip was fun—even the trains and shuttles. Mostly it was fun (and I'm sorry you missed it) to see Betty trying to maneuver that suitcase the size of a house . . . and watch those businesslike train conductors try to shepherd her and the rest of us tourists off the trains so they could keep to a schedule. I don't think those train platforms on the East Coast have a lot of women's groups quite like ours . . .

AGAIN THANK YOU>>>>YOU ARE SPECIAL!!!!!! And please thank John for being such a good sport for moving out of the house for the night.

A note on what's been going on medically since I arrived back home:

I did see my oncologist two days after I got back, and I was anemic from all the bleeding when I was there (by the way thanks for the emergency supplies). It was not so bad, however, that he thought he needed to postpone chemotherapy. I started back on the pump that day, and it was one of the tougher sessions I've had so far as keeping up my energy level—I'm sure it had something to do with starting out tired and I am running out of patience sometimes. Oh well.

He gave me two weeks to recover from the direct liver therapy . . . and then he put me back on systemic IV chemotherapy once a week. I was hoping to be taken off of everything at least temporarily, but he says no. My CEA (Cancer antigen level—it's something produced by tumors) is very slightly fluctuating . . . and that could mean that there is some tumor activity somewhere in my body. This is not unusual, and it appears that Chemo and I are fighting its growth effectively . . . but he says he basically doesn't think it's dead yet so we are keeping vigilant. Traditionally, my CEA levels are not extremely reliable yardsticks, but he wants to play it safe . . . and so do I. Because of hard reactions in the past, he has brought my doses down slightly and hopes that will get rid of the problem without as many side effects.

I saw my internist last week, and I am losing my foot reflexes again—all that means is that I have to pay attention more to walking and balance . . . like the old ladies do. They keep on moving; they just hold railings and don't talk and walk and look around at the same time!!! Not a big deal. I also had a repeat colon exam (I refer to that as the Roto-Rooter service) two days ago to rule out tumor activity in that part of my anatomy. Everything looked good inside, the plumber doctor said, though there is one area of scarring near my original surgery that he biopsied that had a lot of scar tissue. He was not concerned, but they like to be sure. It was around a metal staple, so he took the staple out to give that area a better chance to heal. Can you believe I have staples in THERE???? Apparently, when the surgeon cut out the bad part of my colon he just stapled the ends back together like an old garden hose. I just can't believe they do that—that's like stapling a snake back together. This medicine business just blows my mind . . . but once again, it seems to be working in my favor, so I have no complaints.

David and Liz were both home for Thanksgiving. This was the first time we'd seen Liz since August. She is so happy with school, loves the kids, loves the profs, eats dinner every night at tables reserved for the 45 members (co-ed) of the crew team who come from a three-hour practice on the lake direct to the dinner table (she loves the Jock feel of it all!), and has become involved in a Bible Study weekly in her dorm . . . and once a month all the dorm Bible study groups go off on a retreat for the weekend. She loves the camaraderie and sharing. Sounds like a great school. Their academics are very average, but the self-esteem and religious atmosphere appear to be awesome.

David is doing great. I did go down to San Diego to see him once before Thanksgiving. He and I went to *Phantom of the Opera*. Tony hates musicals (why sing for ten minutes when you can say it in 2 seconds?), and I really wanted to go . . . so when the play came to San Diego, Tony told David he would buy the tickets if David would take me. We had a great weekend. I stayed and watched his fencing tournament the next day and that was really impressive to see. I also did meet my old neighbor from St. Louis, Kathy Brownschidle, who now lives with her three little hockey playing boys and Jack in Buffalo—Kath and her mom were staying at the same L.A. Marriot where we girls stayed last year the night before you left. Tony came down for the day and we stayed overnight, visited until the wee hours, and had breakfast with Kath and her mom before they caught their flight back home. It was great. I smile when I think of her and Jack with three little boys—they're spaced in age just like yours. Busy group! Jack plays Mr. Mom and coaches hockey. Kath is a high-powered exec.

Christine is on OB this month and has delivered 30 babies—advantage of a mostly Mexican county hospital—and loves it! Katie is in Nashville, Tennessee, this weekend interviewing at Vanderbilt Med School and visiting her friend Roger whom she went to Europe with. Tony and I are sitting home alone, playing OLD PEOPLE . . . and savoring the moment. We'll have a houseful in another week or so when the kids return and come home for Christmas . . . and we're looking forward to it. Enjoy a wonderful Holiday with your boys . . . and thanks again so much for the most enjoyable time.

Looking forward to next year . . .

CHAPTER 4

God

Mimi once described her illness as a large boulder that she tried, at first, to push out of her way. Unable to move the rock, she came to see that perhaps moving it was not her task, and she realized the strength she had gained from the pushing. Mimi learned to use her illness as a sort of spiritual 'workout machine' on which she honed her strengths, became her best self, and gave much strength and hope to others—including me.

My mother, like Mimi, lived for many years with cancer before dying at the age of 53. Mom's death affected me profoundly, not just because of the loss, but because her last days were filled with such pain and suffering, and her Christian friends insisted that this was 'God's will.' Angered, I spent ten years after her death as a bitter agnostic. Eventually, seeking reconciliation and peace, I walked into St. Phillip the Apostle Church's RCIA program where, remarkably, Mimi was chosen to be my sponsor. Over the next two years, I had the privilege of learning about God through her eyes, while seeing his love reflected in her. Mimi continued to trust God even while accepting the limits of her humanity—and accepting that we can't always know 'why.' Rather than seeing her illness as 'God's will,' she viewed it as an experience God would help her through and use to create something good. Mimi helped me to see God as a loving companion on the journey of life—a source *not* of pain and punishment, but of *love*, who can help us find joy and strength, while in Mimi's words, we "push [our] hardest on the big boulders of life."

Jennifer Black, M.D.
Friend and hospice doctor

Early-mid-2002

REFLECTIONS IN THE MUD

Mimi tells us again of the power of God and the friends that He gives us.

February 11, 2002

I called my friend Betty in Atlanta for her birthday. She was born on the feast of Our Lady of Lourdes. It was her birthday, but she said that she was sending me a gift. She had just ordered some Lourdes water from the shrine in San Antonio for her sister, Jean, and for me. She 's a spiritual support for both of us in our cancer crusade. Somehow, I felt this gift would be extra special because Betty and Our Lady shared the day. I kept that in my heart.

At Mass later that day, I spoke with Mae Murphy and told her about my friend born on this Feast day. Mae asked if I remembered watching the *Song of Bernadette.* I told her I recalled it from way back in my teenage years, but I don't believe I've seen it since then. She said she had the video and she was bringing it to me. She commented on the powerful drama of the young girl, Bernadette, digging in the mud for the spring of water. I file her comment in my memory. She gives me the video, but it is several weeks before I find the right opportunity to watch it.

Early March

One day when I am especially perturbed about my cancer, chemotherapy, and rising CEA counts, and I am not feeling well. I see the Bernadette movie sitting by my morning reflection chair and decide today would be a good day to watch it. Indeed, I am struck by the scene of the young Bernadette digging in the mud. She is dirty faced, franticly seeking, down on her knees like an animal. I am moved by her simple faith. I am reminded that mine should be the same way.

April

Yesterday the little bottle of Lourdes water sent lovingly by Betty arrives in my mailbox. I placed it, last night, by my bathroom sink. Today is a Wednesday, and I have eight hours of intravenous chemotherapy today. Before I go, I pray for healing of tumors in those areas. I remember how Bernadette of Lourdes washed her face in the water in the movie, but my makeup is already on so I leave my face alone. Off I go for treatment with expectation that the miracle will start to happen . . .

June

Our St. Philip's Pilgrims are traveling this month to the shrines at Lourdes and Fatima with Monsignor. Elizabeth brings Home a bottle of Lourdes water for Amparo. Despite the fact that Amparo's first impulse was to drink the water, she said she wanted to give it to me for my birthday. In my most recent visit with Dr. Patel, we discussed the benefits of considering kidney surgery. I told Amparo that I will save this bottle of holy water from Lourdes and pack it with the personal items I will take to the hospital with me. Amparo's strength of faith will be with me when I go to the hospital. Instead of fear during the night before surgery, I will have the peace wrapped around me.

The week before my birthday I see Irene Sill one day at Mass. She doesn't know that is my birthday, but God does. He gifted me with birth through my mother on that day 53 years ago. This year He will gift me with continuing health. I don't think there are coincidences—I know God has a plan.

Julie Worthing calls just before I leave for Chicago for my family reunion with Christine and she asks if she may list my name in the bulletin. With kidney surgery looming somewhere on the horizon I tell her yes. This will be a big surgery. I will know I am covered by the Church's umbrella of prayers, and it will help me feel secure in my moments of doubt. I will remember how much I am loved and cared about. My name in the bulletin . . .

Early July

The music ministers have now returned from their tour of Rome and singing for the Holy Father, Pope John Paul II. Eileen Lindsey prayed for me throughout the shrines of Europe. I know God heard all her intentions because He quieted the troublesome nerves in her legs and feet and allowed her to go way beyond what she thought she could do. God loves every part of our bodies—He tends even to the feet. "And now God . . . onto Mimi's kidney and lungs . . ."

July 22

Today I see the surgeon, Dr. Belldegrun, at UCLA. He is confident and self-assured. "I can do the surgery," he says. The fear of being "high risk" vanishes when he and I both reflect on the miracle that (as he stated), " You do not look like your history would indicate." I reflect this new confidence based on the reality of the miracles that I have known. I am gaining greater certainty that this surgery is the right choice. August 21 is the day.

By the next day, our family has developed a plan. Tony has the week off. Christine will take a couple days off for the surgery. Liz will try to come down for surgery but considers that it might be more help-ful to take off work time to help me during my first days back home. David will see how he can work out his schedule but will definitely come up during that first weekend of my recovery. Katie, who works there, will always be close by for a laugh . . . or a kiss. I know I can do this surgery now. My pillars are in place.

Later that week

I've been gaining confidence. I'm gearing up for the surgery, probably removal of the kidney. I know I can do it. BUT I have so much to accomplish before then. How to get the house clean? How to get rested up? Find time for prayer and meditation? How to inform every-one I want to tell? Who to enlist as helpers when I'm home on the slower paced—no driving—recuperation track? How to handle chemotherapy this final month while recovering strength? How to fit in a pulmonary consult? A physical? A haircut and dye job? Uh-oh. Worry is beginning to overwhelm me. I can't settle down. I'm restless.

July 26

I'll go pick those peaches before they all fall to the ground. Maybe I'll even make a pie. That'll give me something to do. I'll grab that ladder propped over there under the orange tree and reach for those peaches beyond the roof line. O-o-o-o-f . Not a good idea. The ladder was broken . . . and now so am I. Elbow. Ouch! I have a few mad things to say about lying here in the mud. The sprinklers have recently gone on so I'm a mess of scrapes and blood and mud. I'm just gonna lay here and reflect on how my life has been going downhill lately. I say "sh—" and mean it. Then I start to cry. I feel sick.

God knows I 'm scheduled for kidney surgery, and he knows I'm going to need both elbows to push myself up in bed after my side has been incised . . . so what's the deal here??? I consider this an extremely inconvenient predicament, but O.K., you fallen mud goddess, MOVE!

So I get up and cautiously walk to the swimming pool. My legs hurt. They're bruised, but they work okay. Down the step. Oh, the water feels good on my scraped skin. The mud is washing off. I feel cleaner. I'm feeling bad now about being mad at God. He didn't push me. Then I laugh inside about Monsignor Frost's comment that there is something deeply spiritual and mysterious about Marcia's fall last year. I believe it . . . for her. Now I'm wondering if that applies to ALL falls. Mine? It's just a funny time to think of this. The closest I can come is that by the time I got in the swimming pool I was ready to apologize for the unkind words I had recited while I was down there in the mud. That felt pretty spiritual—the water was cleaning off my body; the apology to God was cleaning my soul.

Then I found out that my elbow didn't work right. So long as I kept it bent and perfectly still next to my body, it didn't hurt. If I tried to extend it or flip my palm up or down, it would hurt a lot. I tried to ignore it and kept it bent and hugged tight to my waist. That's how God holds us when we are wounded. Maybe that was the spiritual lesson.

I walked around the house that night loving my arm. That's all I could to with it. It was pretty useless temporarily. It couldn't pick up things, or even reach up to wash my face or reach down to pull up my pants. I would have to reconsider the things I was currently worrying about accomplishing before I left for the hospital in three weeks.

July 27

Today is Sunday and my arm felt all right to go to church. In fact, all of me is all right. I can't do much except sit and relax. If I rest my arm on the table, carefully, I can hold a pen and write legibly. This is what I've learned since yesterday: Life is so much bigger than the small things we try to accomplish to please ourselves or to feel organized or to meet another's expectations. These next couple weeks before my surgery are not about how much I get done before I go or how well kept the house is when I come back home. Life is about all the people who care and who help me survive through the power of prayer. I think of all the people who have shown care and compassion for me recently, and I am overwhelmed. I often get overwhelmed by this type of loving community.

July 31

Today is chemotherapy time again. Even chemotherapy comes

with its rewards. The nurses are always nice, and Marcia comes with a blender and her special brand of Marcia-ness. I wish I could get organized to spend more time with her, but somehow she has managed to find me (on Wednesdays) when I have no where else to go . . . and she makes those days extra special in a way I can't describe. I no longer think of them as "My chemo days" . . . but as the days to enjoy lunch with Marcia and conversations with Nancy Pelton. It's not where you are so much as who you're with that sets the tone for a day. Marcia reminds me, just by her presence, about how much people care. She's getting ready to go to the cabin so I probably won't see her before I leave for UCLA. She brought me a beautiful card and a hospital present—so many thoughts for me when she has so many concerns of her own. That's what I mean about her special Marcia-ness. Caring.

Random July days this week

Some days I can hardly think straight. Maybe it's because I can't get my elbow to go straight. It seems like my brain lives in my elbow sometimes. Actually, I know that's not true. What's true is the part of the Corinthians message where Paul says, "We are all part of one body . . . when one part of the body suffers, the whole body suffers." That's how my friends and family are. They care. I look forward to the day in the distant future, kidney surgery having been accomplished, when we will all rejoice. I tell people I will be back in Chicago for Gina's wedding on October 5. I see my niece as a beautiful bride. I will do a reading for her . . ." Only these three things remain. Faith, hope and love, but the greatest of these is love."

I am so blessed to be surrounded by so much love. Often, it comes from totally unexpected sources on a surprise day. A couple of days ago in the mail, I received a book from Mary Lue and Janie in St. Louis entitled, *My Happy Heart.* They sent it just because they were thinking about me . . . and wanted to remind me of the Greatest Love of all. I called Richard O'Dell from R.C.I.A. recently because I haven't seen him all summer and wanted to let him know about my surgery. He gave me a lengthy "Richard pep talk" over the phone and came by the next day. (He is surviving a nasty and very rare form of cancer himself.) Richard loves to share. He wants me to be blessed with the same returning health that he is blessed with. Also, just out of the blue one afternoon recently, Mary Devereaux called to say she wanted to give me a statue that a nun brought back for her from Medugorje. Faith.

That is what I see in all the people who care so much. Love. That is what I feel for all of them. So many kindnesses. Great and small.

August 1

Mary Richard called a couple days ago to see if we could still meet for lunch today. My answer to her a couple days ago was "Mary ,I love to go to lunch with you anytime." . . . and I get up this morning knowing that it will be a lovely day. Mary is one of those women with the authentic gift of hospitality. Despite the fact that she has recently kissed her sick mother and placed her eternally into the hands of God, helped Dana cope with the sudden loss of her mother, and is now trying to help Cammie and the rest of the Harrisons through their tragic loss, Mary is gracious as usual. She has the added attraction of Lauren and Nick for lunch today. It's simple to see they love her as much as she loves them. Her serenity is a stabilizing force for these teenagers who have to face another of life's harsh realities.

Mae Murphy has joined us today for lunch. I knew she was coming so I made sure to bring along the video she lent me six months ago, *The Song of Bernadette*. I tried to write her a thank-you note in which I would apologize for the lack of speedy return. She didn't care—lending movies and sharing spiritual encouragement is her business. She flipped the returned video into Mary's purse so Mary could take it home to enjoy and learn from. Mae, by the way, I did learn a very special lesson from the video . . . and I also think there was "God's timing" on the return of your video:

Last night I placed the video in my purse so I would not forget it when we went to lunch. I then proceeded to the bathroom sink to get ready for bed. Visions of Bernadette washing her face in the muddy waters of the underground spring came to my mind. I saw my little bottle of Lourdes water from my friend sitting in the corner of my bathroom counter.

Healing—that's what was happening to my elbow. Like Bernadette digging in the mud, I too had begun this week in the mud , only mine was on my back under the peach tree. The message of the mud lives on. Have faith, child. Come wash, and be healed. Yes, my elbow was the small reminder I needed to remember that God will continue to heal. Now when I get nervous about this upcoming kidney surgery, all I need to do, Mae, is wash my face . . . and smile at the faith I see looking back at me from the mirror . . . the reflection of eyes that can see God's blessings to me in His Love manifested in the kindnesses and prayers of friends. Thank you, my friends.

Early-mid 2001

OUR HANDS, OUR HEARTS

*This is a series of reflections that Mimi wrote during a particularly hard time.
It again speaks to the power that God had in her life.*

Early March 2001

"It's all right, Mary, except for my hands . . .
They burn, and my fingertips are throbbing
from the chemotherapy and the radiation . . .
I don't sleep at night. Blistering hands keep waking me up."

"Well, Mimi, sometimes the Healing Touch of God
can feel like that . . ."
The words penetrated. Silence.
And I saw in my minds shadow, the face of my friend—
A smile reflecting a knowledge in her heart of Love,
her deep blue eyes glistening of familiarity with God,
blinking and blending her tiny tears of compassion,
mingling her understanding of pain with mine.

Mary, Mary . . . which Mary was it?
The voice on the phone was the Mary I know,
but the smile and the eyes, the knowledge, and the pride
in the power of the Son . . . came from a depth
even beyond the telephone's end.
There was so much power, such clarity in the words—
Were they spoken in a chorus of voices?
Was it also the voice of my other friend Mary
who would live with Jesus soon?
Or my Godmother Mary who, like you,
also blessed me with a Nativity?
The suggestion, the assurance, the faith in the healing power of God
sounded as though it originated from one
who had held the very Hand that healed.
Was it Mother Mary who led little Jesus by the hand,
and later caressed the bleeding hand of her Son
and Savior of the world?

All my Mary's are special gifts . . .
All my Mary's are "the song."
You, from your heart, began the single note,
carried forth from the Holy Spirit . . .
which created a whole orchestra to burst forth from my soul . . .
and keep on playing.

My hands are no longer an encumbrance, but a reminder . . .
Thank you, dear Mary . . . they are wrapped in song . . .

Written with Love to Mary Richard

August 15, 2001

Lately I've been overwhelmed by the deaths of so many friends, many from cancer . . . and I feel like the roll call list is getting shorter and shorter . . . and I'm still on it . . . almost seven years now. Seven years . . . Larry Wolf recalled to me his dream of the seven flower pots falling from a ladder. "Seven," he says "is the perfect number." It is God's number denoting completion . . . and then the phone call came from the hospital room where his beautiful daughter Michelle had completed her life on earth. I understood the meaning of the seven . . . for Michelle.

But what does seven mean for me? Is it Completion as Michelle had received . . . or perhaps for me the completion of active disease? Is seven years later when I will attain remission? I don't know what seven means for me. I don't usually try to figure it out, but I remember Betty Bova called from Scottsdale soon after Easter, and we got into one of our philosophical discussions about the trials and successes of my seven-year disease. We both recognize that my life is made of many miracles . . . and she good humouredly remembered that she'd heard sometime ago that the human body has a very major change every seven years. Perhaps my change could be freedom from cancer. We both decided that was a fine idea. Betty's discussion gave me cause to pause . . . and believe once again that her remarks didn't come out of nowhere. Could they have been delivered from the Spirit as a message of hope for me? I know God helps us when we are down . . . and I'd been feeling pretty down . . . perhaps especially noticeable because of Tony's stress related depression surrounding the death of his mother in January . . . and my accumulated exhaustion from . . . so many different things.

Palm Sunday, April 8, 2001

A gathering of friends in the evening after church,
A pot-luck dinner and a thoughtful exercise.
Another Mary
Mary Lou and I are assigned as partners
Alone in a room I tell her of my frustration—
the limitations of living with cancer.
"I want to do so much more with my life," I say.

"Who do you envy?" she asks empathetically.
"No one." I say, "Because nobody has everything I want . . .
a lot of people have some of what I want,
I'd rather just know all of them and learn little pieces
from each person
Nobody has it all.
There are no perfect people.
Only Jesus is perfect."

"Close your eyes now, relax, get peaceful," is Mary Lou's invitation to me.
I do it. I like the quiet. I am in a comfortable place.
"Is anyone there with you?" says her gentle voice
that makes me think.
I look behind my eyelids and smile . . .
I don't see anyone, but I feel . . .
"Yes," I say with certainty and awareness.
"Jesus is here with me . . . He's always here . . . why do I forget
to see Him?"
I want to cry. I'm angry with myself. I've kept Him waiting, I
often do . . .

"Can you take Jesus' hand?" Mary Lou gently guides . . . "Can
you reach it?"
"Yes." (I feel it near)
"Will you do it?"
"Yes." I will reach for the hand of my friend.
"How does it feel?
"Nice." I say with warmth enveloping me, "He's PERFECT."
I don't let go.

"What is separating you from what you really want?" Mary Lou asks Us.

"Worrying about my disease. Being limited by it." I say alone.

"I want to build on my present and walk into my future . . . and not see a finite end . . . and not be tired . . . and not be afraid."

"How are you limited? What's holding you back?" asks Mary Lou . . . or is it Jesus asking?

"It's . . . a . . . w-a-ll," is my slow answer to the questioner.

"What's the wall made of?" the gentle voice asks.

"It's made of . . . numbers. They're my cancer counts. I see them now, just numbers.

They are real, but they are fake. They are true numbers, but they can give me a false sense of who I am. The numbers are fake . . . I just *think* they're real.

"Is the wall real?"

"Yes, but it's plastic." I answer in close-up-observation-astonishment, "like Plexiglas. It's only a **plastic** wall!" I can see **through** it. I'm fine on the other side of the wall!" I say with excitement . . .

"But, I just can't get through it **now**," I say with some sadness.

"If you hold Jesus' hand, can you go through?"

"Yes, He can go through anything. He can bring me with Him . . . through the wall." The certainty in my own voice surprises me.

"We can walk right through it together.

I knew that all the time.

I just never asked Him to hold my hand.

I never reached my hand out.

I was so DUMB."

I opened my eyes as I became aware that the voice was my own, berating myself .

Then I remembered the patience of the Shepherd, and answered

"All I have to do is ask Him now . . ."

as we walked through the wall together hand in hand.

I am crying now at the table where I sit, because I am happy inside the wall.

We just went through the wall.
I'm in the safe part now, holding onto Perfection.
Jesus is laughing, it's a smile laugh.
He told me so many times that was all I had to do.
I don't know why I didn't do it. I didn't think about it.
He is just smiling, softly laughing at me. He knows how silly we are.
People are just silly
We can be so dumb.
Jesus is laughing at my silliness because he knew that I knew what to do all the time.
I just didn't do it. I don't even know why.

Mary Lou is laughing and crying with me. She says that all the years I've been sick, I've been doing the things that were most important to me. She saw with eyes of Another what my own eyes often did not see . . .

Thank you, Mary Lou, for reaching out your heart to me so I would reach out my hand . . . to Jesus.

Good Friday, April 13, 2001

Two days ago, one doctor discontinued my continuous chemotherapy. Seven weeks was all I could have right now. A second doctor said the inflammation of my fingers must be controlled so I am taking large doses of Prednisone, which disrupt my ability to sleep . . .

I cannot sleep on that medication, so I went to church to pray
It was Good Friday, a time for reflection, so I stayed all day.

The first meditation was "The seven last words of Jesus"
As He looked down from the Cross where I know He sees us.

But the Outdoor Stations of the Cross I could not do.
Instead I sat alone exhausted on the front church pew.

And I whined to Jesus that my fingers hurt so much,
Then remembered the way Mary had said, "Jesus' Healing Touch . . ."

My mind moved to Mary's mentioning how during Holy Week she cried

For the sins of man that caused Our King, Lord God to be crucified.

There were glistening tears of sorrow clinging now on my eyelashes
As I looked up at hand-carved Jesus, draped in red and purple sashes.

I stared at His carved hands—one reached down in love
while the other rose in power . . .
Then His Holy Hand reached down for mine as we sat together
in that hour.

I could not place my hand in His,
though comfort I was needing—
For my hands were only blistering;
His Precious Hands were bleeding.

And so I took His Hands in mine
and caressed them for His comforting,
So guilty, so desperate did I feel just then
to relieve His suffering.

Jesus and I sat together as His Peace
penetrated the distress I was feeling,
And His Hands were pressed upon my heart—
The Reality of Healing.

I knew Mary was right about "God's Healing Touch" when I felt Jesus
hand on Good Friday. Thank you, Jesus, for this affirmation of your
Love.

April 27, 2001

Why is it that we wonder so about the messages that come from
God?

I think it's because as adults we so often fail to believe with the
simple faith of a child.

By late April I was beginning to recover from most of the side
effects of the chemotherapy/radiation combination that I had received
in March. Last year I had missed participation in the Relay for Life, but
this year I was involved again. On the Friday night before the Saturday
Relay, I was out on the field at Cal State helping the staff set up the
CBCC booth. Debbie was there with her little daughter Madison who

shared with me that she had no doubt that God had laid "His Healing Hands" on me . . . because that is the way she prayed . She said it in a simple sentence. I thought about her lesson for weeks . . .

Madison has her own story. I wrote it about her . . . but mostly to remind myself. It's included at the end. I hope you'll read it and enjoy my magic moment with Madison.

May 21, 2001

By May I knew with certainty that God had touched me with "His Healing Hands." I began to understand once again that He had indeed been doing this for me all my life. Lately, I had needed more affirmations . . . and He had given them to me regularly. Another affirmation occurred when I attended as Amparo's guest the Carmelite Rite of Formation at Christ the King Church. The Mass with Monsignor Frost officiating was filled with the Joy of the Holy Spirit. I had never seen this priest but had heard highly rated reviews from Marcia, Amparo, Mickey, and others. He must be fun, I thought . . . though I was not prepared for the simple humility, humble servant hood, honest sincerity, and holy anointing, which I received on the steps of his church. He told me he has known of me from Marcia, and he prayed for me as he placed his hand on my head in blessing. As I had seen him hug the children during communion, I thought these must be the same type of healing hands that little Madison imagined resting upon her dolls at night. As He placed His hands upon me now, I knew that his prayers played a part in my healing.

July 27, 2001

Marcel waited for me after church. She has a small, white, embroidered handkerchief given to her by a friend who has been to Medugorje. She wanted to pass the kerchief on to me. I took her gift and carried it in my chemotherapy pump pouch. I know beyond a doubt that Marcel's prayers, along with the united prayers of our Christian community, and the examples of faith in all who believe have helped me. Her gift affirmed what I already knew, and what my blood tests are currently confirming—that I am being healed.

I hope you realize, my friends, how much your prayers, affirmations and messages of love help me to daily grow stronger in my faith. With God all things are possible.

Feb. 1996

Mimi shares again her reflections on writing.

February 5, 1966

Critique for Mary Lou:

My husband and I took off a couple days and drove up the coast Highway 1. I was trying to work on my book while we were gone, but I was more inspired to help you work on yours . . . I enjoyed visiting with you last week and discussing our respective works. Thanks for your tips on trying to develop my story as a series of smaller books. That gives me more freedom.

Anyway, I just finished reading the copied workshop notes you gave us and noted the one suggestion to WRITE whenever possible so I figured I would write this. By the way thanks for all those notes . . .

Following were my ideas:

We were alone on a high, vista point overlooking a beautiful beach on the coast somewhere north of Hearst Castle. We were watching and listening as the waves crashed violently on the massive rocks to our left. Yet on the right of this same scene was the babbling of a brook so quiet in comparison that it seemed like a summer space. The only uproar there was where the brook turned to a waterfall easing down over the rocks before shooting outwards and upwards over an upturned rock like a powerful fire hose spraying into the ocean. Between the two scenes of crashing rock and quiet brook were dozens of sea gulls circling in the air, some drowsily and some determined, as they dropped down for dinner into the dark water.

I wished you were there to see it. It reminded me of the many small scenarios in your mountain scene meditation. It made me think that you could write a full book on meditations of nature—a mountain scene (and definitely your Mt. Whitney reflections), a meadow scene, a beach scene, a street scene, an office scene, a church scene, a home scene, and a grandmother scene. (It was nice to meet you and Dana at the Convention Center baby shower.)

I was thinking that I should have been contemplating how my own book would unfold, but this scene was not conducive to contemplating how to organize. So I free floated within my head instead, and I asked God why I was thinking about you . . . and I got this cute answer from somewhere: No one lives in a vacuum . . . you go to a group session . . . and the group becomes a part of you . . . your ventures become joint ventures . . . different people attract different people . . . kind of like He put magnets in each one of us . . . to attract different people at different times . . .

Also that question we spoke about that day in your office. Do the stars also reflect the sun as the moon does? I asked Tony that on the drive home in the dark and he says no, actually the stars are burning all the time, hotter than the sun. I thought to myself: Well, those are busy little buggers then. The stars are individual performers, burning, burning, burning, allowing God to place them into constellations for our amusement and astronomy. When we are busy we are like stars. The moon, on the other hand, is still (as we should be sometimes) and reflects the light of the sun. How about tying that in with this passage from 1 John 3:2–3 where it says we will unite with God in the future and "we shall be like Him (perfect reflection) because we shall see Him as He really is." I love that passage.

I hope to see you on Wednesday, but I have a big chemotherapy treatment on Monday . . . so I might not be friendly . . .

Summer 2002

SIGNS, WONDERS AND MIRACLES

*This was written in 2002. Betty Greene was her BSF leader and a friend
who died after a long illness. Again, this story speaks of her reliance
on God and the comfort she received from the words of the Bible.*

After finding out last week, May 23, my CEA had risen from
19 to 29 in one month, I moved up my scans by two weeks. Tony was
at the office, but the scans could not be pulled up off the computer so
we walked down to the CT screen to look at them. There are more lung
tumors and the existing ones have grown. The kidney tumor is larger.
I'm stunned but calm. Tony seems ok.

The following week Girish reads them out. I see his reports.
Advise follow-up . . . and gradually it starts to sink in. Ravi is still
away in the middle of his five week journey. I am seriously beginning
to wonder if this last course of Cisplatin and 5-FU has done any good
at all. My white counts have been down in the 2,000 range since the first
week, and now it's week nine and they are still low. We have reduced
the dose to the point that I'm wondering if it's even worth doing. I
don't know where to go for advice.

Things came to an emotional head when I was contemplating
a trip back to Chicago, but I felt my immune system would be at risk,
and I worried that I would just be postponing needed chemotherapy
and further tests. I am constantly exhausted, it seems, just thinking and
worrying about all the "ifs." When I try to call and speak with Dr. Cartmell, I get Annette in triage. I tell her I am trying to decide whether
or not to do chemo this week or cancel it. She asks me if I'm trying to
choose quality of life vs. quantity of life. "Not yet," I tell her. "I'm just
wondering about next week! Would a week off maybe help build my
white cells?"

I'm disturbed after this phone call. That is my reality. I'm the
one who has to ultimately make those decisions. I feel isolated and
alone. I'm sad. I'm scared. Christine is helpful. She helps me confront
my realities. She says, "Dr. Patel would say 'Live a little. Take your
trip.' " She will come with me to Chicago, rent a car, hotel, whatever is
necessary to make me feel comfortable and get rest while I see my family. She is patient. She is kind. We will go.

Tony gets hold of Dr. Cartmell for me. Alan says to come and get chemo, but he'll look over the chart and maybe lower the dose. Some chemo is better than none . . . and we will stay with this one until another plan of action is decided upon. I feel more secure.

On June 8, the Feast day of the Sacred Heart of Jesus, I woke up and did the Living Faith meditation chapter. It eased my fears and put me back at ease. Do not be terrified, it said. Adoration before the Blessed Sacrament that day was soothing.

In addition, I had been thinking much of Betty Greene lately, how she must have felt as her lung fibrosis was diagnosed and worsened. Every once in a while, I saw her smiling at me and sometimes she said with the Wisdom look' mm-hmm . . . and you think God is saying NO. This passage seemed to come from God. I can reflect back to it and get calm. It recalls for me so much of our final study with Betty on signs, wonders, and miracles.

The reading: Deuteronomy 7

When the LORD your God brings you into the land you are entering to possess and drives out before you many nations . . . , seven nations larger and stronger than you- and when the LORD your God has delivered them over to you and you have defeated them, then you must destroy them totally. Make no treaty with them, and show them no mercy. Do not intermarry with them. Do not give your daughters to their sons or take their daughters for your sons, for they will turn your sons away from following me to serve other gods, and the LORD's anger will burn against you and will quickly destroy you. This is what you are to do to them: Break down their altars, smash their sacred stones, cut down their Asherah poles and burn their idols in the fire. For you are a people holy to the LORD your God. The LORD your God has chosen you out of all the peoples on the face of the earth to be his people, his treasured possession. The LORD did not set his affection on you and choose you because you were more numerous than other peoples, for you were the fewest of all peoples. But it was because the LORD loved you and kept the oath he swore to your forefathers that he brought you out with a mighty hand and redeemed you from the land of slavery, from the power of Pharaoh king of Egypt. Know therefore that the LORD your God is God; he is the faithful God, keeping his covenant of love to a thousand generations of those who love him and keep his commands. But those who hate him he will repay to their face by destruction; he will not be slow to repay to their face those who hate him.

Therefore, take care to follow the commands, decrees and laws I give you today. If you pay attention to these laws and are careful to follow them, then the LORD your God will keep his covenant of love with you, as he swore to your forefathers. He will love you and bless you and increase your numbers. He will bless the fruit of your womb, the crops of your land-your grain, new wine and oil-the calves of your herds and the lambs of your flocks in the land that he swore to your forefathers to give you. You will be blessed more than any other people; none of your men or women will be childless, nor any of your livestock without young. The LORD will keep you free from every disease. He will not inflict on you the horrible diseases you knew in Egypt, but he will inflict them on all who hate you. You must destroy all the peoples the LORD your God gives over to you. Do not look on them with pity and do not serve their gods, for that will be a snare to you. You may say to yourselves, "These nations are stronger than we are. How can we drive them out?" But do not be afraid of them; remember well what the LORD your God did to Pharaoh and to all Egypt. You saw with your own eyes the great trials, the miraculous signs and wonders, the mighty hand and outstretched arm, with which the LORD your God brought you out. The LORD your God will do the same to all the peoples you now fear. Moreover, the LORD your God will send the hornet among them until even the survivors who hide from you have perished Do not be terrified by them, for the LORD your God, who is among you, is a great and awesome God. The LORD your God will drive out those nations before you, little by little. You will not be allowed to eliminate them all at once, or the wild animals will multiply around you. But the LORD your God will deliver them over to you, throwing them into great confusion until they are destroyed. He will give their kings into your hand, and you will wipe out their names from under heaven. No one will be able to stand up against you; you will destroy them. The images of their gods you are to burn in the fire. Do not covet the silver and gold on them, and do not take it for yourselves, or you will be ensnared by it, for it is detestable to the LORD your God. Do not bring a detestable thing into your house or you, like it, will be set apart for destruction. Utterly abhor and detest it, for it is set apart for destruction.

1996

PERSONAL BLESSINGS FROM THE
HEALTH CARE MINISTRY

This shows the importance of faith in Mimi's fight with cancer.
It also shows her thoughtful nature.
In the midst of her struggles, she sat down to
write this note of thanks to those that served her.

I never fully appreciated the Health Care Ministry of the Church until I needed it myself. When I was diagnosed with metastatic colon cancer two years ago, I was unable to reach out to embrace the church, but the church came to me. While I was recovering from colon surgery in the hospital, the appearance of members of my faith community was like a soothing balm on the rough edges of my emotional pain. They reassured me that God had not forgotten me and their example reminded me to pray. The love of God, which they displayed, helped me overcome my fear and doubts; their prayers encouraged me to offer prayers of my own that gave me a sense of peace in these troubled times.

After I returned home from the hospital, it was wonderful to have one of the Eucharistic Ministers come to my home on Sunday with Holy Communion. That helped me focus on The Lord's Day and not just one more of My Days on the slow road to recovery. My battle has not ended yet. I have returned for at least three major surgeries and have been anointed and blessed by Father John. That process and the accompanying prayers have sent me off to surgery confidently knowing that God blesses me while I sleep . . . and when I wake, those Health Care Ministers will be there as a constant reminder. May God bless all those who care.

-Mimi Deeths

July 2001

FAITH

Mimi's friends often times asked her to write to friends of theirs who were facing cancer.

July 18, 2001

Dear Susan,

I talked to my friend Rose Cinquemani last night, and she asked that I pray for you in your new diagnosis of metastatic breast cancer to your brain. I'm so sorry to hear that news because I know it fills you with fear, and probably downright frustration and anger that you have to go through more tests, more treatments, and more inconveniences instead of moving forward with your life as you've planned.

In human terms, I think we'd all agree that life is difficult enough—without all these frustrations and fears we have to deal with. When we are struck by a **second** occurrence of cancer, life may seem downright unfair. Once is difficult enough. Why twice? I speak from experience because I've been there, Susan . . .

I was diagnosed with colon cancer, already metastatic to my liver, seven years ago, at the age of 44. In that first year I had a colon resection—a second abdominal surgery to place an indwelling catheter for chemotherapy directly to my liver. A brain tumor was discovered, and I underwent brain surgery. I also had a liver resection with cryo-surgery (freezing of tumor) to my liver at UCLA. I remained on chemotherapy throughout the whole year. (And yes, what Rose said is true—I remain still on it seven years later. The whole thing is a mystery and a miracle . . .)

I did not see at the time of diagnosis how a human body such as mine could survive. I had a weak constitution in courage, a general lack of discipline, and low tolerance for pain. I grieved for the people I would inconvenience and disappoint—mostly my husband, children, and my 75-year-old mother. Good friends from my Bible Study Group came by and reminded me that God was with me and God could sustain me. That, indeed, the God who created the universe could certainly take control of my disease. This I have found out with each passing year is the truth of all our lives upon this earth.

God has helped me beyond any expectations I had of Him. In

my cancer experience, He has taught me how BIG He is when I am frail and weak. I pray that He will display Himself to you in the same way.

God's primary prerequisite is that you have FAITH. Just put yourself in the loving hands of God who created you. I found that is not hard at all if you believe these words from Psalm 139:

O LORD , you have searched me and you know me.
You know when I sit and when I rise;
you perceive my thoughts from afar.
You discern my going out and my lying down;
you are familiar with all my ways.
Before a word is on my tongue
you know it completely, O LORD .

You hem me in-behind and before;
you have laid your hand upon me.
Such knowledge is too wonderful for me,
too lofty for me to attain.

Where can I go from your Spirit?
Where can I flee from your presence?
If I go up to the heavens, you are there;
if I make my bed in the depths, you are there.
If I rise on the wings of the dawn,
if I settle on the far side of the sea,
even there your hand will guide me,
your right hand will hold me fast.

If I say, "Surely the darkness will hide me
and the light become night around me,"
even the darkness will not be dark to you;
the night will shine like the day,
for darkness is as light to you.

For you created my inmost being;
you knit me together in my mother's womb.
I praise you because I am fearfully and wonderfully made;

This became one of my favorite Psalms right from the beginning of my diagnosis. Each time I recovered I knew more deeply that I am indeed fearfully and wonderfully made. So are you. These words remind me that a God has control over my life. I only **thought** I was the one in control. Can you imagine how much easier it can be when we let God take charge of our sick body? It allows us to trust the doctors whom God has prechosen for us at this time. Trust is important. Try to remember to pray for the doctors who treat you. I like to think of the physicians at CBCC as servants of God. In my dealings with them I have found them all to be strong men of faith who work hard to control cancer and blood diseases, and they have been made humble before God because they have seen the horrible devastation and power of disease, yet strive with their God-given talents to bring cancer under control for the betterment of mankind. I think they are doing what God expects of them with the talents and personalities He has given them

Recently, Susan, I went through six weeks of radiation with Dr. Desai at CBCC. It was just this past March, and the treated area was my left adrenal gland. Originally I had a choice of either radiation or surgery. I prayed that God would give me peace with my decision. As I fell asleep that night, I recalled a passage from my Bible that I looked up the next morning. I share this passage with you:

> Rejoice in the Lord always. I will say it again: Rejoice!
> Let your gentleness be evident to all. The Lord is near.
> Do not be anxious about anything, but in everything,
> by prayer and petition, with thanksgiving, present your
> requests to God. And the peace of God, which tran-
> scends all understanding, will guard your hearts and
> your minds in Christ Jesus.
> Philippians 4:4–7

Upon meeting Dr. Desai, I was immediately made **aware of his gentleness** in manner. My son made me laugh when I told him about this passage in the Bible helping me be at peace with my decision to do radiation. He said, "You're right on that one, Mom, radiation is peaceful (compared to surgery) . . . **and it certainly transcends all understanding** because you don't understand a thing about how radiation works. (He knows physics is not my strong point.) I felt affirmed. I progressed through radiation with no problems. Three months later I can say it appears that the radiation was successful in knocking out that tumor.

I know Rose told you that God loves you and will care for you through this trial, and she reminded you about the passage in Matthew. It is the beautiful one where God tells us not to worry about ourselves for He clothes the birds of the air and the flowers of the field. How

much more even must he care for us? This passage is in Matthew 6:25–
33, and I would recommend reading it . . . and believing it.

In addition, I offer these passages from the gospel of John:

> "Do not let your hearts be troubled. Trust in God ; trust
> also in me."
> John 14: 1

His words are for all time—that means he says the same thing
to us today.

Later as Jesus prepared to depart, knowing that the Holy Spirit
would come to help us after Jesus went to heaven, he said these word
of promise:

> "All this I have spoken while still with you. But the
> Counselor, the Holy Spirit, whom the Father will send
> in my name, will teach you all things and will remind
> you of everything I have said to you. Peace I leave with
> you; my peace I give to you. I do not give to you as the
> world gives. Do not let your hearts be troubled and do
> not be afraid."
> John 14:25–27

I hope, Susan, some of these words will come to life for you. Try
reading them when you are afraid . . . and hear them as coming from
the mouth of God. Believe them, and they will sustain you through
the fears and inadequacies you may feel. Be courageous and call upon
the Lord. Be courageous and call upon your friends and family to help
you. Drugs and radiation may temporarily affect your ability to think
clearly and confidently, but allow yourself to fall back into the loving
arms of God your Father and trust Him to direct your steps back to full
recovery.

Call me if you wish. I'm usually home after 2 P.M. and free until
about 5 P.M. when my husband gets home.

1997

BIBLE ON THE BUN

*Again, in this story, we see how simple faith can make all
the difference in how one deals with a diagnosis of cancer.*

I first met Dorothy about a month ago. She was a tiny, little woman, frail but spirited, accompanied by her big, burly husband who praised her proudly as "my wife of forty-three years and the mother of our six children." Dorothy was scared. She had recently undergone bladder surgery. The diagnosis was cancer. She had a stoma to deal with; that whole concept was new and annoying. In addition, she had undergone her first sessions of chemotherapy and as she said, "Lordy, they had made me so sick. I just didn't go back for anymore."

I worried about Dorothy. She didn't seem to understand the system. In dealing with cancer, you just have to do things you don't want to do. In fact, I think you have to grow to really hate the disease so you'll work even harder to fight it. You have to accept the surgeries; you have to endure the chemotherapy; you have to learn to be patient and to trust. You must trust your physicians, and beyond that, you must put your faith in God.

Dorothy was a fighter, but I was afraid she had given into the confusion and complexity of a medical world that was overwhelming to her. In the weeks following my first meeting Dorothy, visions of Dorothy popped into my head during quiet moments, and then I saw her again. We were at a cancer support group together. She looked much stronger and seemed not so scared. When the group was asked if they felt faith played a part in their coping with cancer, Dorothy willingly spoke up.

She related an incident where, "Oh, that right BUN was so sore. It hurt so bad. I took my Bible and I put it there right under my bun, and I was healed! Slept that night through like a baby, kept that Bible under my bun!"

I laughed when I heard the story; I laughed when I even thought about the story. That night I awoke in my sleep, and the story was right there like a video in my conscious mind. When I woke up next morning, the story came back.

I got in the shower and as water and shampoo dripped from my hair, I understood why I was silent last night about my own faith experience. So was everybody else. Dorothy's faith experience, shared so simply and so openly, left the rest of the group in wonder and awe. We are all grappling with an intellectual, emotional, and rational exercise in faith. We wonder with the "Why me?" mentality. We are struggling with the place of God in our lives. Hopefully, we are drawing nearer to our compassionate and merciful Lord as we cope with this disease called cancer.

Dorothy's experience was so profound that it caused us all to pause. Dorothy is not struggling to find God. She's been alive a long time. She knows Him. No doubt, she's seen Him at work as she and her husband raised their family. God's Word is close to her, so close that she knew immediately where to turn in her time of need. Perhaps therapy or medication or merely the passage of time would have cured her as well, but what she chose was wise and wonderful—the best in alternative medicine for those who have a child's trust—The Bible on the Bun.

> People were bringing little children to Jesus, to have Him touch them, but the disciples rebuked them. When Jesus saw this, He was indignant. He said to them, "Let the little children come to Me, and do not hinder them, for the kingdom of God belongs to such as these. I tell you the truth, anyone who will not receive the kingdom of God like a little child shall never enter it." And he took the children in His arms, put His hands on them, and blessed them.
> Mark 10: 13–16

Mid-1996

MOSAIC OF LOVE

*Mimi wrote this after her birthday in 1996
and intended it to be a chapter for her book.*

Thank you , Ladies, for making my birthday special. It was wonderful to share the day with you all at Susan's house. The potluck luncheon was exceptionally good . . . beginning with Carol Ann's gazpacho, through all the delicious and healthy vegetables, rice and black beans, and stir fry dishes, and ending with not one—but two of Carolyn's delicious deserts—lemon meringue pie and German Chocolate cake . . . and those chocolate-covered Rice Crispy treats.

(I always like when there are as many desserts as anything else.) We really must do this again sometime . . . whose birthday is next?

I appreciate all your gifts, and I will think of you each time I wear my angel pin, put on my T-shirts, look at my Monterey Bay seal, view my hips where the delicious See's candy has been deposited, look at my picture frame and magnetic plaque, and settle into the soothing sounds of Carey Landry's music. Everything has special meaning for me.

Mostly, however, I am happy that you could all be there to celebrate with me. Your friendships, prayers, and our celebration of FAITH have meant so very much to me especially during this past year. I praise God for ALL his interventions in my life and for placing you around me to be my angels and my friends. God bless you all!

As I read over my cards, I saw the beautiful mosaic of friendship and love and caring displayed in your specially chosen verses, Scripture, and music. I want to share all of these with you . . . since God has given his Word to all of us. Following is my gift to you all:

"For he will command his angels concerning you to guard you in all your ways. "
Psalm 91:11
from Mickie and Ashley
from Francine

"And surely I am with you always."
Matthew 28:20
from Brooke who brings great happiness to me and to the deaf man at the nursing home with her sign language skills

"'I know the plans I have for you' "declares the Lord' 'plans to prosper you and not to harm you, plans to give you hope and a future.'"
Jeremiah 29:11
from Carolyn and Susan

"If the LORD delights in a man's way, he makes his steps firm; though he stumble, he will not fall, for the LORD upholds him with his hand."
Psalm 37: 23–24
from Carolyn

"Praise be to the God and Father of our Lord Jesus Christ, the Father of compassion and the God of all comfort, who comforts us in all our troubles, so that we can comfort those in any trouble with the comfort we ourselves have received from God. "
2 Corinthians 1:3–4
from Elise

"Praise be to the God and Father of our Lord Jesus Christ, who has blessed us in the heavenly realms with every spiritual blessing in Christ. For he chose us in him before the creation of the world to be holy and blameless in his sight. In love he predestined us to be adopted as his sons through Jesus Christ, in accordance with his pleasure and will—to the praise of his glorious grace, which he has freely given us in the One he loves. In him we have redemption through his blood, the forgiveness of sins, in accordance with the riches of God's grace"
Ephesians 1:3–7
from Susan

"I was at the point of death, my soul was nearing the depths of the nether world;

I turned everyway, but there was no one to help me. I looked for one to sustain me, but could find no one. But then I remembered the mercies of the Lord, His kindness through ages past;
For he saves those who take refuge in Him, and rescues them from every evil.
So I raised my voice from the very earth, from the gates of the nether world, my cry.
I called out: O Lord, You are my Father, You are my Champion and my Savior;
Do not abandon me in time of trouble, in the midst of storms and dangers.
I will ever praise your name and be constant in my prayers for you.
There upon the Lord heard my voice. He listened to my appeal. He saved me from evil of every kind and preserved me in time of trouble.
For this reason I thank Him and I praise Him; I bless the name of the Lord."   (NAB)
Apocrypha
Sirach 51: 6–12
from Amparo

There's a very special angel
Who has nothing else to do
But spend each moment day and night
Just watching over you

Hallmark Card with angel pin
from Amparo

"The Lord bless you and keep you;
The Lord make His Face shine upon you
and be gracious to you:
The Lord turn His Face toward you and give you peace."

Numbers 6: 24–26
Prayer of Moses
from Betty

"Love is patient, love is kind. It does not envy, it does not boast, it is not proud. It is not rude, it is not self-seeking, it is not easily angered, it keeps no record of wrongs. Love does not delight in evil but rejoices with the truth. It always protects, always trusts, always hopes, always perseveres.
And now these three remain: faith, hope and love. But the greatest of these is love."
1 Corinthians 13: 4–7, 13
from Irene

. . . . There, now, I have another chapter for my book. Thanks for adding so much to my life. I hope you like these verses. I do. Please don't just keep them for yourself. Share them with friends, especially when they are sick or feeling sad. Believe me, it will really lift their spirits.

July 1997

FIGHT BACK

Mimi was always helping of people diagnosed with cancer. This is a letter written to her cousins after Gus was diagnosed with cancer

July 10, 1997

Dear Donna and Gus,

I'm sorry I have not contacted you sooner. I had intended to give you a call after your presence was sorely missed at the Twin Lakes Reunion. It was only then that I found out about Gus's cancer. I wanted to cry—it is a nasty disease. I know you have discovered that already. I spoke with Tom at the lake, and he says you've already gone through the radiation phase of treatment and had begun the first session of chemotherapy, which left you feeling nauseous. I can empathize. I hope your doctor or clinic prescribes good antinausea medication—that's what has allowed me to survive chemo for three years.

The most common antinausea is Compazine. I tried that—it works for some people, but it didn't make a dent in what I was feeling. I was then given Ativan, which is a stronger antinausea with a mild antianxiety agent in it (admit it, we deserve it—a disease like cancer should make anybody a bit anxiety ridden). Donna, you might like some of that too! I know cancer is about as hard on the other family members as it is on the patient. I found that the advantage of Ativan is that it can make you more relaxed and allow you to sleep easier. I generally sleep for about 20 hours almost straight through on the day after my weekly treatments. It's sort of a lost period in my life, but at least I'm not living in the bathroom! I do have a water bottle always by my bed, and I sip it whenever I can—one thing I have learned to appreciate is to force fluids. I ended up almost delirious in the hospital once because I thought I was too sick to drink—even if it's an eyedropper full at a time, you've got to find a way to get that water down. Lots of water also protects your kidneys from cell destruction due to the potency of the drugs your body is being loaded with.

There also is a relatively new drug for nausea. Its name is Zofran—supposedly it works right on the barf center of your brain to make you not feel nausea. The main drawback is that it is outrageously expensive—about twenty dollars a pill, three times a day! If you have good insurance, this is a great medication. It is worth a try, however. If it works for you, it's worth the money. When I need them, I can usually limit myself to one or two days a week so the cost is not too bad. Sometimes the doctor can get you samples from the drug reps. Learn to be bold and ask about all this stuff. I have learned to be nice but very assertive.

When I was first diagnosed three years ago, my oncologist told me that although my prognosis was poor, he had an arsenal of drugs and treatments and surgeries that could be tried. In addition, he said, there is DAILY new information coming to him over the computer. He said there is always hope . . . if I would just bear with him and take ONE DAY AT A TIME. That's a hard concept for most of us to handle. We like to plan our lives . . . now is the time to reduce life to small increments, very valuable increments. It's a time to focus in on yourself and your spouse . . . and let the rest of the world go by. You can catch up later. It takes energy some days just to be civil to the people you love, but it's worth the time and energy. Hang in there together—you will learn to appreciate one another more than you ever thought possible . . . and you'll spend a long and wonderful life together after this treatment phase is all over.

It does end even though it may not feel that way while you are in the thick of it. Though I have not had the exact same treatments as you, I have three women friends who have had the same lung/brain combination you have. All three of them are doing or have done three, eight-hour-a-day treatments in a row followed by a twenty-one day rest period. One has been in remission for two years now. One is feeling normal after four courses, and there is no further sign of tumors three months later. The third is still in treatment being encouraged by the other two. I have come to know these women through cancer support group, which I have been attending for about six months. Cancer support group might be something you may want to consider at some time. Some people find it beneficial; some find it overpowering. I find it to be both—I like the information that flies forth. It's good to know that other people experience the same things you do—agitation, nervousness, sleeplessness, "hyper" reactions, highs and lows of emotions, fear, and anger. It's good for me to know my reactions are "normal." I am, however, sometimes overwhelmed because cancer is so prevalent and hits so many young people and disrupts their lives so much. It hits so many old people and leaves them with no energy or will to fight back. It's a mean disease, but . . .

Donna and Gus, WE ARE BIG ENOUGH TO FIGHT BACK.

Disruptive cells should not be allowed to take over our bodies, our minds, or our souls. We have people to love and support us. When we love them back, we will fight to keep that love growing. We have our faith, and whether we have actively practiced or not, God watches over us just the same. He loves even the lost sheep. He waits with His arms open wide to bring back any of those who have wandered from the fold. All we have to do is seek those arms. If your faith is not strong now, just repent (turn back) and go to those welcoming arms. That's where I always return in my moments of insecurity. I have come to feel God's presence . . . and to tell Him how wonderful He is to create a world so incredible and to fill it with people who love me. I tell Him I want to stay, and He has let me. He'll do the same for you. Have Faith.

There are a lot of resources you'll be pulling from the next several months. Good doctors will put their heads together on your behalf. Nurses will care for you. Your family and good friends will be your supports through love, compassion, and understanding. Your response and attitude will determine your will to survive. Your faith can allow you to ascend beyond the nitty-gritty aggravations of this disease. I'll be praying for you and thinking about you both. I know you can do it! I have.

I have enclosed several books written by Richard Bloch. Richard was diagnosed with lung cancer in his forties. I met him two years ago and have even received personal replies to my letters to him. Two years ago he celebrated his 50th wedding anniversary to Annette . . . and this man was not supposed to live for three months. I believe his books speak for themselves. They helped me immensely in my early months of coping with cancer. I hope they will help you as well. I have purchased many copies, and I pass them on gladly to friends. Richard will send free books if you ask . . . for yourself or friends.

You and both your families remain in my thoughts and prayers. I would like to keep in touch with you. Sorry I did not call you when I was in Chicago a couple weeks ago. Mom was not feeling well after her surgeries and I was tending to her, trying to see all my siblings, and getting her in to see her internist and surgeon. The week just went too fast. Hope your rough periods fly by just as quickly . . .

Aug 1998

ANSWERED PRAYER

This was written to Mimi's friend's sister. Jeanne and Mimi fought very similar battles with cancer. They were born within a month of each other. When one was having more trouble with cancer, the other was too. When one got better, the other did too. Mimi and Jeanne died within two days of each other and their funerals were on the same day and at the same time, given the time change.

August 17

Dear Jeanne,

I have intended to write this letter for over a month, but I have not had the discipline. I made a concerted effort to play to the maximum this summer and invite too-long-out-of-contact friends over to swim and just use every opportunity to have fun!

Unfortunately, my oncologist raised my chemo dose at the end of June—and after five weeks at the high dose, I was pretty toxic and had to have a three-week body rest. I had terrible burning and painful hands, feet, and burning eyes and insides for a week. The second week was better. By the third week, I made a ten-hour round trip and spent a night with my kids down in Southern California and attended my niece's first National Junior Women's 20 km bike race. That was a first for her and for me. It was fun.

It was a challenge to accomplish all I did in one weekend. Tony did not want to go—too rushed—but I felt a great sense of accomplishment . . . and of course, the added bonus of seeing my son and daughter at school.

I talked to Betty just before she came to visit you last week . . . and was excited to hear that the tumor killer cells were rising. I pray it keeps up. I know it is relatively disappointing to hear that you'll probably be there for another month (miss the beginning of school, miss family, impatience with the "program," seemingly slow progress, etc.) but, you've invested so much already in your recovery that I view the extra time as just a stronger guarantee.

I know you feel like a pincushion with the daily injections, but it sounds like they are producing the desired results. I knew they would—but again, we must work on God's timetable, not our own. I hope you have gotten some rest and enjoyed your visits with the family as they have all taken turns to fly over. I'm sure you feel as I do that God could not have blessed you with a better group of family and friends. The support is tangible and very lingering and extremely dear.

I have been involved in a neighborhood ladies Bible study this summer, and I have enjoyed meeting new neighbors and appreciated the discipline of keeping me in the Word. I am leading this Wednesday's lesson, and there is emphasis on God answering our prayers. I appreciate the assurance and want to share it with you this week. Following, are the verses that I am discussing.

Perhaps the best known is this:

Ask and it shall be given to you;
Seek and you shall find;
Knock and the door will be open to you.
For everyone who asks receives;
He who seeks, finds,
And to him who knocks, the door will be opened.
Matt 7:7–8

Further reinforcing the above truth is this verse from
1 John 3: 21–22.
Dear Friends,
If our hearts do not condemn us,
we have confidence before God
and receive from Him anything we ask, because we obey His commands and do what pleases Him.

Also from 1 John 5:14–15:
This is the confidence we have in approaching God:
That if we ask anything according to His will, He hears us. And if we know that He hears us—whatever we ask—we know that we have what we asked of Him.

Another from the Gospel of John is this:
If you remain in Me and My words remain in you,
ask whatever you wish,
and it will be given to you.
This is My Father's glory,

that you bear much fruit,
showing yourselves to be my disciples.
John 15:7–8

Jeanne, I really liked this lesson because it reinforces my asking mode. God does not mind being bombarded by our requests provided we do it with the right heart attitude, with confidence, and with the intention that we will go on to bear much fruit as His disciples. I know you do all of these things. I pray that you continue on in confidence and faith . . . and may God grant you your request for continued good health.

It sounds like you are getting some much needed rest over there in the Bahamas. All that helps in fighting cancer and building your immune system. I am trying to strike a happy medium in that regard. This summer I have really worn myself down . . . but I have enjoyed it! I'm sort of looking forward to the cooler weather and more indoor time. My letter writing and book reflections have pretty much been on hold—and I miss that soul-search work.

Speaking of soul search—I have just finished a book I think you would really appreciate. It made the Bestseller list recently and is called *Tuesdays with Morrie* by Mitch Albom. It tells the story of a sociology professor who befriends a student, Mitch Albom (the author), when he is a young man. Years later as the old professor is dying, he calls upon Mitch to finish the final thesis by teaching him through the final stages of life. The beauty of the book is that the professor reveals to Mitch what he has learned is important in life. It's a heartfelt and truly sharing project, which makes for wonderful reading. I think it would be a good reference for your Death and Dying class at Fontbonne. I liked Morrie. He reminded me of my own father whose name just happened to be Maurice. I'm sure you will see your own father in Morrie also—Betty always talks so lovingly of him.

I hope your family is doing well and that the newlyweds are happy. I'm sure they all look forward to your return to St. Louis. You'll be there soon and the homecoming will be wonderful . . . but for now, just keep working on those cells!!!!

Early 1998

GOD IS IN CHARGE

This was written to a friend when he was strug-
gling with a diagnosis of cancer.

January 18, 1998

(Sorry, that's when I began this letter. It is now Feb. 5, as I finish—lots has happened in that three-week interval. My attitude has healed—your calling upon me to help Susan was one step in that healing process. Enclosed are some of the daily reflections (Spirit gifts) which have helped me. I share them with you since I think our physical/fear concerns of recent weeks are similar.)

Dear Jeff,

Thanks for telephoning last week. I hope I was able to encourage you in the midst of your concerns. Actually, I was in the pits myself . . . and as usually happens, in trying to encourage someone else, I brought more joy unto myself. I was affirmed in my efforts by the readings at Mass the following day (or maybe two days later) and yesterday and today as I was reading my Bible Study notes, I was again blessed by encouragement for all of us—Tony and I, you and Berniece.

Here are my reflections:

I woke up and began the day with reading the little pamphlet I have called Living Faith. This was the first thought that struck me. We may be bruised because of our conditions, but God understands and sympathizes with us . . .

The reading from Samuel 4:1–11 reminded me that I had forgotten to bring God into my daily life. The focus lately has been on me and my uncertain condition and the sometimes seemingly insurmountable problems I have to work through. I forgot that GOD IS IN CHARGE.

When the Ark of the Lord's Covenant came into the camp, all Israel raised such a great shout that the ground shook. (This is what we should be doing because the Lord's covenant is WITHIN US—we should be shouting for JOY, not worrying what the next cancer marker level will be.)

Now there happens to be a nasty turn of events in this biblical account, the Israelites who had the ark in their midst were defeated by the Philistines. That didn't seem fair, but I believe what I was to learn from this is that, like those Israelites, I must not be content with just knowing that God is in me. I must speak with Him, consult Him, and truly believe that He is in control. That's what the Philistines did—though they were pagans, they had respect and fear of the Lord. *When the Philistines learned that the Ark of the Covenant had come into the Israelites camp, the Philistines were afraid. "A god has come into the camp," they said. "We're in trouble!"* The Philistines then proceeded to rout the Israelites and capture the Ark of the Covenant. The Philistines had faith that this God could strengthen them. They were willing to fight (even harder than the Israelites) to bring God into their midst. I realize that I need to WANT FAITH so badly that I am willing to fight (pray actively, seek Him with my whole heart) to overcome my enemy (fear).

Psalm 44 tells about the power of God to control the fate of nations at war. If He can do that, surely He can command these piddly, little cancer cells in our bodies. Listen to some of the truths in this Psalm:

> We have heard with our ears, Oh, God, our fathers have told us what you did in days long ago. With your hand you drove out the nations . . . It was not by their sword they won the land. IT WAS BY YOUR RIGHT HAND, YOUR ARM, AND THE LIGHT OF YOUR FACE FOR, YOU LOVED THEM.
> Psalm 44:1–3

> I do not trust in my bow, my sword does not bring me victory; but you give us victory over all our enemies, you put our adversaries to shame.
> In God we make our boast all day long.
> Psalm 44:6–7

> We are brought down to the dust; our bodies cling to the ground. Rise up and help us; Redeem us because of your unfailing love
> Psalm 44: 25–26

Feb. 5 continued . . .

Need I say more, Jeff? I feel in my heart that this lesson is meant for both of us. That's why I feel compelled to send it. We need to remember that FAITH in the midst of our physical seekings. We still need our doctors. I feel God put them there for us—they are his tools. We must remember to pray as we seek their guidance. The Spirit is waiting to be asked to help us in our daily lives.

I keep you in my thoughts and prayers. Enclosed is a copy of the letter I sent to Susan. I enclose it because I want to share the woman's story (biblical) also with you.

I've also been receiving great insight from my Bible study ACTS and letters of Paul, so I end with his greeting . *May Grace and Peace be with you, Berneice, and all those whose lives you touch.*

Sept. 2000

THE KINGDOM

Mimi loved God and took advantage of every opportunity to share the good news with others.

September 28

Dear Judy,

Now that I'm home from vacation, enjoying the cooler, fall weather, I'm trying to sit down at the computer and recall the highlights of my summer. It's sort of my quarterly letter to myself . . . so I can remember what was and is important.

One highlight definitely is the day we spent at your and Jim's new home in Caliente. What a lovely, peaceful place on earth, and it was so meaningful to me to be able to spend it with friends, those I have known for most of my years in Bakersfield, and the new ones I have met and enjoyed so much—like you!

Now I don't remember if I wrote you a thank-you note after that day or not. Sometimes, I do things in my postchemo haze brain, and I do not recall ever doing them; other times I doze with drugs, and I dream that I have organized and accomplished the nitty-gritty duties of the day. When I wake up, I find I have not accomplished them at all. In a way, each day is a new surprise!!!

Fortunately, I do have days of high perspective, and I would have to venture to say that they are probably accentuated by the frequent days of quiet reflection that have became a necessary part of my life.

One of those days of heightened perspective was this past Tuesday, during the funeral Mass for Marci Tivnon. I saw you and Jim there, along with so many others who came to celebrate her life and honor her family. I could not help but to be most joyful for Marci when I heard that she had called upon Father Craig Harrison in the final months of her illness. "Ask and it shall be given; seek and you shall find; knock and the door shall be open to you," is an invitation spoken by Jesus.

Several times during her illness I had written to Marci imploring her to seek God, if she had not already done so. Others must also have been encouraging her in that direction, for as Father Craig stated, she had asked for him to come. As her body weakened, I believe she came to realize that none of the earthy possessions mattered—and only Love remained. Love of her family, love for her friends, and love of God.

I felt like Marci was sending a closing message to us all. I know she was your friend. Out of a strong sense of emotion, and also a sense of duty to God who has sheltered me, I want to feel that you have been invited to explore a deeper relationship with God. I know your depth, your goodness, your gift of easy laughter, your pride, and your love for your family and your friends, your kindness, and your appreciation for nature. I know how much you have been blessed with and how very appreciative you are. It was delightful to see your new home and the loving regard you have for all God's creatures and the awesome beauty of nature all around you.

I have always appreciated God's gifts to me, and I'm sure Marci did also. What I have come to realize primarily through my cancer experience, and what I feel Marci came to seek during her terminal phase of cancer, was a genuine relationship with God. He longs for us to talk to Him and know Him. He gives us so many, and although He wants us to enjoy and appreciate the gifts, He wants also for us to appreciate more deeply the Giver. When we give a gift to a friend, our hope is that the friend will enjoy the gift, but don't we really give the gift as a promise of an even deeper relationship with that friend? The gift itself is incidental—what matters is the growing relationship of warmth, love, and respect and joy between the giver and the gifted. As we want that bond with our friends, God wants that bond with us. This we need to remember.

This letter may sound presumptuous to you. If it does, I'm sorry. That is not my intent. I just have felt a need this week, in working out my emotions following Marci's funeral Mass, to invite her friends and my friends to open their hearts a little wider to let God in. I just want to say that if you ever want to ask me any questions about God, Jesus Christ, or the Holy Spirit, I will do my best to answer them for you . . . or refer you to someone who can.

We can all see God's majesty in the wonders of his Creation. In the first chapter of the Bible, we are taught that God created the world in six days, and He proclaimed it "very good." We, too, should see it as very good and protect it. Then on the seventh day God rested. That seventh day is our Sunday, our time to rest with God. Only if we allow this can we build up a relationship with our Creator. He has already given us the beauty of his world, now he wants to sit with us , like a good teacher, on the seventh day (really every day) . . . and teach us more about Himself.

Creation is only one facet of our Almighty God. He wants to show us His other qualities in order to help us gain an even greater depth of appreciation for who He is. His faithfulness and unconditional love are revealed in the second book of the Bible, Exodus. His laws, protection, covenants, and blessings for his chosen people are revealed in Leviticus, Numbers, and Deuteronomy. The Old Testament history goes on to show the failures of humanity and the ever present faithfulness of God.

The New Testament teaches us how God sent his only Son into the world to save sinful man and a sinful world. We have the teachings of Jesus and the creation of a new covenant that can bring us eternal life if we believe that Jesus Christ died for our sins. The New Testament is filled with encouraging messages that we should build up the Body of Christ (the Church), and that we should bring the Word of God to those who hunger for it.

God has so much in store for us that we cannot even begin to contemplate. I hope that Marci has approached the entrance to this mansion that Jesus teaches about in the gospel of John 14:1–4 where He says to his disciples,

"Do not let your hearts be troubled. Trust in God; trust also in me. In my Father's house are many rooms; if it were not so, I would have told you. I am going there to prepare a place for you. And if I go and prepare a place for you, I will come back and take you to be with me that you also may be where I am. You know the way to the place where I am going."

I believe that Marci did know the way. She has traded in one mansion for another Mansion. This one is eternal. I know she wants to greet her family and her friends there in a future time known only to God. In the meantime, we can all come to realize more deeply how special the gift of life is. Knowing God can make that gift even more precious. This knowledge is what I would wish most to give my friends.

Please think about this. In the meantime, I will keep you in my prayers. Enclosed is my prayer for you.

1996

PRAYER BREAKFAST

These are Mimi's reflections on a prayer breakfast that she went to.

Dear Amparo,

Thank you for the tickets to the prayer breakfast. Stella and I had a wonderful time, but we were sorry you couldn't come . . .

We got there late because I lost my car keys and hunted all over the house for them at 6 A.M. I did find them and when we arrived at the filled auditorium after 7:00 A.M., everyone was already seated and eating breakfast. An usher waved us up to two empty seats in the SEC-OND ROW. Guess who was introducing the program at the Speaker's platform?? Edith and Gary Gibson. Edith did the introductions—she was marvelous. She sends her love to you.

Following the breakfast, Edith introduced the first speaker, Stanley Simrin. He is a devout Jew and quoted Moses' last speech to the people and one of your favorite quotes from Isaiah, "I saw the Lord not in the earthquake or the wind or the fire, but in a still small voice."

Michael Fisch, a city leader, prayed next for leadership for our city's leaders. He asked that God may give the city leaders guidance and wisdom, and that they might understand and put into operation the golden rule "To do unto others as you would have them do unto you."

Next there were three beautiful praise songs sung by the 60 member chorale group from West High School. Our own Leta Sage from BSF was the pianist, and she looked beautiful in her formal black dress.

Then came the senior class president from West High School who asked God to bless the youth of our city, to keep them from being led astray with the allures of the world. He prayed for the parents, who model for their children, and for the teachers, who influence the minds of their students. He was a stunning example of leadership for our young people.

Steve Perez then read Psalm 23 and focused on the line "He leads me beside still waters" and explained it in a way that made me hope Betty Green was there listening. He told of the Shepherd and sheep. Sheep are afraid of any rippling water. With their heavy coats and bulky bodies, they know they will drown. Even though people say sheep are dumb, they instinctively know they can't swim. The good shepherd always looks for still water before he leads his sheep to drink. If there are no still waters, the shepherd waits 'til the sheep are sleeping, and then he fashions a rock dam so that the water will not move in that area . . . and the little sheep will not go thirsty. How this reminds us of our God . . . who protects us and guards us even as we sleep. He understands our limitations and works with them. He understands the weight we carry on our shoulders and protects us from out fears.

At this point Edith introduced the main speaker for the program, Alonzo McDonald. He is a wonderful man. (Stella talked to him after the program and he lived very close to her home in Massachusetts and knows her little town!) Mr. McDonald was introduced with his credentials including an M.B.A. from Harvard and having served on the White House staff under President Jimmy Carter. He was a very humble man. He began by saying that he felt he did not even have to speak that the program thus far had been so inspirational that he felt he would not even have to speak, yet the audience could go away satisfied! He's a good praise person.

He did speak, however, and it is clear to me that he has put into practice the goals in the book we have read, *HALF TIME* by Bob Buford. He began his speech by saying he was in awe of the Spirit, invoking the Spirit to guide his words, and he prayed for forgiveness for the unworthiness of the speaker (himself). He went on to say that we are pilgrims searching for meaning of Life. This is due to four trends he sees in the way society is today. First, there is a void in our lives. We are guilty of one thing that Ecclesiastics warns us about, " Beware of chasing the wind." We do that; it's futile—there tends to be a God-shaped vacuum in the center of our lives . . . The second problem with our society is the fact that most of us have no real friends. We all need a true friend with whom to search, someone who understands life's priorities and will sit and talk about things Spiritual. Thirdly, ours is a doubting society. We need to develop FAITH to counteract this shortcoming in our lives. Faith is vital. Doubt is not the opposite of Faith; doubt is a part of Faith. Lastly, he said we are a society disillusioned with our worldly possessions and goods. These things have not proved to be as satisfying as we hoped they would. He said he is lucky; he has accomplished much in his life, and he is more satisfied than most. He has been blessed with many gratifying jobs, but laughingly, he says, "he never stays in a job very long." People call him a good "bouncer." He is successful in business; he loves interrelating with people.

Mr. McDonald went on to say that our lives are sort of like a mountain climb. We spend so much time and money training to climb the mountain. We spend a great deal of energy to get to the top . . . and once there, we stay for a very short time only . . . and the descent begins. He referred to that great parable of the workers in the vineyard who came to work in shifts, but when pay time came along, they all got paid the same amount. Well, he says this is not good economics, nor is it good labor relations, but it is a wonderful parable because it is evidence of the GENEROSITY of GOD.

He further stated the we need to LET GO, LET GOD.

His five suggestions:

1. Pray and reflect.
2. Read Scripture.
3. Memorize key verses for lonely times (hotel rooms at night, etc.).
4. Seek silence and solitude . . . in order to LISTEN to God.
5. Develop a Spiritual confidant—a search of classical literature will show this has been done since earliest times. Socrates, it is said, spent time in seeking the TRUTH. Plato said that friends were more important than performance of deeds . . . Victor Frankl, a survivor of Auschwitz, says LOVE is all that matters. Leo Tolstoy, a great Russian novelist, warns against selfishness, greed, and ambition.

The thoughts expressed in the paragraph above, Mr. McDonald says, are difficult for a man like him, a negotiator, because negotiators are used to getting things. He says he needs to remember to ask for the Holy Spirit's guidance that He may pour out love and be of service, as stated in Philippians, "with humility." Keep in mind John 12 . . ."Love one another" and Isaiah 26 . . ."Keep in perfect peace. Be steadfast." Finally, remember the beautiful quote of wisdom from Proverbs 3 . . ."Trust in the Lord wholeheartedly. In all thy ways acknowledge Him, and He shall direct thy paths."

Following this main speaker, our mayor, Bob Price, responded with gratitude to the day's messages and prayers for our city of Bakersfield.

The closing prayer was delivered by Bernie Herman of the Hospital Association here in Bakersfield. I want to write and ask him for a copy of his speech. I'd like to incorporate some of what he said in my book. He quoted Matthew 6:33 . . . 'But seek first his kingdom and his righteousness, and all these things will be given to you as well.'

He then talked briefly about M. Scott Peck's book, _Pathways With A Heart_. He talked about the argument some people offer that our God cannot be both compassionate and omnipotent for therein lies a contradiction in suffering. If God were omnipotent, He would prevent suffering. Therefore, he is not compassionate. If God is truly compassionate, He is not omnipotent, or He would not allow suffering. What these people fail to realize, perhaps, is that our OMNIPOTENT AND COMPASSIONATE GOD may be challenging us. He (God) has left it to us to fulfill our highest potential. If we do this, WE will be able to relieve suffering in the world.

There were some awesome thoughts expressed this morning. I've tried to capture them for you. I'm sorry you missed the Prayer Breakfast, but thank you so much for getting the tickets for Stella and me.

CHAPTER 5

Melody

Mimi shared her testimony. God is still kind and loving to me. Mimi's optimistic way of life, her unfailing strength, and her steadfast faith are my goals. I have to charge onward, fight caner, live everyday, never give up, put myself in God's hand. GOD HAS HIS WILL.

Melody Kuo (12/13/54- 1/18/2001)
Friend and fellow cancer patient

2/25/1998

When my mom got cancer, I really didn't know any other people with cancer. I was definitely a bit naïve back then. Mimi let me see another side of cancer. She showed me that you could live with cancer. She was so encouraging. She gave us all hope—hope for the body, but more importantly, hope for the spirit.

I will never forget when I visited Mimi when I came home for winter break in 2003. I had no idea that Mimi's condition had gotten worse. My dad and brother came to pick me up from the bus station and one of the first things he mentioned was about visiting Mimi. To be perfectly honest, I didn't want to go. I had just gotten off a bus from LAX and a 10+ hour plane ride from Japan. I just wanted to go home, but I'm so grateful I went to see Mimi. Although she was physically weak, her spirit was strong. I can only pray to be so steadfast and strong. It's funny how we think we're going to cheer up people, but they end up cheering us up. We think we're going to give them hope, but they give us hope.

It makes me sad to think I didn't want to go. How selfish of me. Mimi showed me just the opposite. She showed me how selfless people can be. I used to think that people nearing death would have mostly selfish thoughts, but both Mimi and my mother taught me otherwise. When I get a headache, I want the world to stop, but both of these amazing people were just so genuinely concerned with others. It is truly amazing. She didn't complain about her condition. Instead, she praised her family and God. I can still picture her face lighting up as she talked about her daughters. It's something I'll never forget.

If it's true that you die the way you live, Mimi lived a life full of grace, humility, and joy.

Kendon Kuo
Friend and Melody's son

Early 1998

NOTES ON TALK TO CHINESE LADIES

Through a friend from her children's high school days, Mimi got involved in the lives of the women from the local Chinese church. One of their members had cancer, and Mimi was asked to give a talk to them in order to help them learn how to help their friend. These are her notes from that talk in 1998.

Asked to deliver my testimony—notes—keep it short and on track so you will have time to ask questions. I want to address your concerns.

Four years ago, 45th b-day, healthy person becomes sick. Prognosis was week or months (I did not know this or acknowledge this publicly though I sensed it and researched it; my family knew—so we did not openly discuss it).

New experience for all of us. Little in life had prepared us to meet this crisis. We had to take it one step at a time. I set my goal to be present at the graduations of my three daughters, nine months into the future. I would do all in my power to make it!

My route to acceptance was Faith—only thing that helped me make sense out of what had happened. Their way of handling me was with Love and Patience. Immediate family took care of my needs. Bible study and church friends prayed and helped me maintain my faith. Friends did practical things for me—shop, errands, carpool my kids, doctor visits.

This allowed me to use my limited energy resources for things that were meaningful and necessary for me at the time. Rest, read, visit, prepare simple meals and sense that I was still useful, though even in a small way. (Merlene took me to my daughter's basketball games.)

Doctors tended to my physical needs for treatment, pain medication, and anxiety and nausea medication when necessary.

First year—colon surgery, placement of porta catheters, two angiograms, brain surgery, liver surgery, chemotherapy weekly, multiple MRI's. By the end of that first year, we were making some headway—beginning to get a hold on the disease. Beating the odds. I was cheered on by this thought . . .

I tried to be dressed, with make-up on and hair combed so I looked good. Looking good makes most of us feel better. I liked people to say I didn't look sick—that made me feel like I didn't have to be sick.

Second year—continued chemotherapy because CEA (cancer antigen) was rising. Took almost a full year to find the tumor that was forming. It was in my adrenal gland. Took much detective work to locate it. Surgery was difficult. Lung surgery is excruciatingly painful and uncomfortable recovery.

Third year—maintain chemotherapy for one year and then hope to be in remission.

Fourth year—nine months ago, wean slowly off chemo (joint decision based on the facts we knew between me and my oncologist). I did not feel I could continue weekly doses—it was a quality of life issue for me. Hard decision, began counseling to help cope with the frustration of reentering into mainstream society. Family issues, emotional ups and downs, what does the future hold for me????

I am dealing with that right now—Remember it has taken nearly four years for me to do this. Do not expect that your friend can grapple with these issues immediately. Be patient. Give her space.

Values of counseling. Not everyone needs this or wants to participate in it. I was not concerned with counseling in the early years of my illness. I did not think I needed it. As I continued to deal for three years with my disease, I got impatient and frustrated. I tried counseling and found that it helped me to unload burdens with an objective listener. My husband is loving, but he wants to "fix" things. Some things in life just can't be fixed quickly. This was leading to some frustration and lack of communication with my husband. Neither do I want to share all things with my children—they have their own lives to live. I would prefer to recognize my problems and do some sorting out for myself (with counseling help: this can be with a professional or a trusted friend) THEN after I have done some of my own mental homework, I am better prepared to discuss my problems and concerns with them because some of the emotional frustration has been dealt with already.

I currently live WITH my cancer. I recognize and accept it as a chronic disease

(not so different that any of the other chronic diseases that people must live with—this attitude helps me have less self-pity.)

I see chemotherapy as a necessary medication though with many side effects. I have some control. I choose to live with the side effects because I WANT TO LIVE.

What does living mean?

On my good days I do as much as I can.

On the bad days I allow myself to be lazy.

I don't feel that I have to offer excuses for the way I feel.

I try to eat and exercise wisely—I only have one body to serve me, this way I will get maximum performance from my body.

However, when my body shouts that it has a craving for junk food or that it does not want to go for a walk today, I usually excuse it. (I like to think of myself as a "permissive parent.") I will let my doctors and psychologist tell me when I need to discipline my body. Although my body has Cancer, it is only a small part of me. I still like my body so I try to be nice to it . . . most of the time.

I surround myself with positive, encouraging people. I deserve it.

I do not have to put up with people who don't understand me or who "bully" me and assume that I am not trying. These kinds of people discourage me and harm the mental attitude that I have been working so hard to create.

I try to see another center of the universe besides myself. I reach for a goal, a dream, an achievement, God. I try to do things that will help others. This gives me a goal in my physical life. I try to seek a God—this is a goal for my emotional and Spiritual Life. I read about Him (my Bible), I listen to music that soothes (reinforces strong emotional feelings like love and peace and beauty) I reflect on positive feelings and on God (silence and teachings of others), speak with Him (in both talking and listening Prayer). I recognize Him as the Creator of all.

By building a personal relationship with Him, I am learning to trust Him to guide my life. This can remove much of my anxiety and fear.

What I share with you, about how I handle my disease and cope with it, is not very much different from the way all you good people handle your own life crisis whatever they may be. I am telling you just to encourage you to think harder and to realize that Melody's needs for all these things are intensified at this time.

I know you want to help her. Here are some practical ways that I have found useful.

Early 1998

HOW CAREGIVERS AND CONCERNED FRIENDS CAN HELP

This is the list that Mimi gave to her Chinese friends when she spoke with them on how to help their friend with cancer. It can be used as a guide by anyone.

I compliment you on how you have already begun to help Melody. You have shown you care by the attention you have given Melody and her family. You are taking time to educate yourself on some of the ways of coping with cancer. You are praying for her. Sometimes when I was very sick, I could lie in bed and feel very grateful that good friends were praying for me—there really was nothing else they could do for me at the time. Prayer helped to increase my feeling of security and gave me HOPE.

Chiu-yee has requested that you send cards, call on the phone, and drop in, and share a pie, a cookie, a joke, a story, and your presence. These are all wonderful ideas. I enjoyed all of these things when I was sick. It let me know that people cared. However, there were times when I was too sick to appreciate any of these things. Please be aware that there will be times and days when Melody will only want to rest and be alone. Her body is going through a difficult process of chemotherapy, and rest is very important. When any of us are sick, our bodies need to rest. Respect her need to rest during the day—ask her what hours might be best for her today. Don't stay too long if she is tired.

As Melody gets used to the chemotherapy schedule, she will have a better idea of what days she will feel terrible and what days she will feel good. Try to plan a little luncheon or a day out for her on one of her planned, good days. This will give her something to look forward to while she gets over the rough days. If the plans do not work out, be hopeful—maybe tomorrow or next week will be better.

Melody needs to get through one day at a time right now, and she does not get to go out very much. Try to bring the outside into her home. Share favorite tapes or CD's, books, magazines, articles—these things she can use at her own pace when she feels all right. They will help remind her that you care.

Help Melody see the good things in life—one of my friends kept a journal of good things. She would not go to bed at night until she had at least one good thing to list for that day. It made her notice the small things in life that meant so much—an act of kindness, sharing a cup of tea with a friend, a meal prepared and shared with her family, a friend to walk around the block with, a glimpse of her son turning into a young man, her husband's quiet understanding and patient love.

Help her find laughter. Doctors say humor is helpful in healing. Norman Cousins, author of *Anatomy of an Illness* writes the following: Some people , in the grip of uncontrollable laughter, say their ribs are hurting.[1] The expression is probably accurate, but it is a delightful "hurt" that leaves the individual relaxed . . . It is the kind of "pain" that most of us would do well to experience every day of our lives. It is as specific and tangible as any other form of physical exercise. Though its biochemical manifestations have yet to be explicitly charted and understood as the effects of fear or frustration or rage, they are real enough.

BE COMPASSIONATE. I recently attended a spiritual retreat dealing with the topic of compassion. Compassion was defined as "walking with feeling." You cannot take away the pain, and you can not let yourself be totally drawn into the pain, but you can:

BE THERE beside the person(s) suffering.

LISTEN TO THEM. Realize, that at this moment, life has taken a turn that is difficult for them to understand and work with. They are puzzled, overwhelmed, and confused. Your listening without judgment will help them work out their difficulties.

HELP THEM BE INCLUDED AND FEEL UNITED AND VITAL even though they may not be able to fully participate in life's activities to the extent that you are. Phone calls, visits, cards, meals, and other acts of kindness will help them feel included.

A SUGGESTION TO FRIENDS WHO ARE HESITANT TO BECOME INVOLVED because they "don't know what to say" or what to do or how to act. Relax. Do the best you can. Years ago, I did not know how to approach a friend whose child had cancer. So I made dinner for the family and dropped it off at their home. My heart was beating fast, my knees were trembling, and I felt sick by the time I rang the doorbell. I wanted to cry. Then my friend came to the door. She welcomed me in. She cried as she hugged me. I cried with her. SHE was the one who gracefully made ME feel comfortable as she apologized for letting HER feelings show. My discomfort with the whole situation dispersed immediately in that moment—we were both mothers, both friends, and now we openly showed the truth that we both had feelings. The tears were healing. I challenge you to try it . . . I have a feeling Melody and her family have the grace to make you feel comfortable. They need your compassionate effort and understanding. You will grow, too, in the richness of the relationship.

> *Be completely humble and gentle; be patient, bearing with one another in love. Make every effort to keep the unity of the Spirit through the bond of peace.*
> *Ephesians 4:2–3*

March 1998

CONNECT

This is a letter that Mimi wrote just prior to giving this talk to her Chinese friends.

March 11, 1998

Dear Brother Bede,

Thank you for the beauty of the mission you have been presenting at St. Philip's. One of the glimpses I have seen of God's glory, since you gave us the assignment to look for these everyday miracles, is this: I shared in the funeral of Norman Gibson this morning and saw a family lovingly say farewell to a man who is going where he belongs now. The glimpse of Heaven touching earth has seldom been more poignantly displayed to me.

Then I stayed for your mission on how to show compassion, and I heard God speak to me through you. He said just what I needed to hear in order to put events in my life together, to become more whole again, to be "connected" as you said. Your words helped me put finishing touches on a presentation, which I am to give on Saturday evening this week.

I have been asked by the Chinese American community here in Bakersfield to come speak to them, present my personal testimony on living with cancer, and make suggestions to them concerning how they can best help a Chinese woman in their community deal with the devastating cancer diagnosis she has recently received. I have never spoken publicly on this topic before, but I am with several of these Chinese Christian women in a non-denominational Bible study and had the true heart conviction that I must honor their request to speak with them. Several of them have walked silently beside me as I have battled my own cancer for the past four years.

I have been shown the compassion of which you spoke today— be there, listen, incorporate the experience into your life. My friend, Amparo, (with whom you spoke on Tuesday) was my strongest personal ally, confidant, and compassionate friend. In addition, I had the wonderful family support of my husband and four children and many friends. I was blessed with a combination of doctors and support staff filled with God's wisdom.

Nearly four years ago, I was diagnosed with colon cancer metastatic to my liver. My surgeon and internist believed I had two weeks to two months to live. My oncologist, my family, I, and God had other ideas concerning the length of my life. Through seven surgeries, including brain surgery, more than three years of continuous chemotherapy, painkilling, anti-seizure, and anti-anxiety drugs, emotional fluctuations, periods of doubt, and eight months of psychological counseling, I have become closer, as you said, to God's perfection. I know I still have a long life to go in order to improve still much further toward that goal.

Being compassionate will be a step in aiming toward that Perfection, and I will attempt to introduce the Chinese community to this concept, this virtue. In addition to telling them about the physical reality of cancer and its treatments, I want to add how they can be emotionally supportive of their suffering friend. I look forward to sharing with them how the compassion of which you speak can help unite all of them together.

Thank you for your very wise and timely words. I thank you and the other monks in your community for the many thoughts you have shared with us. I try to take them into my daily life. Enclosed is an article I wrote over a year ago following Father Dan's advent mission here where he asked us to come up and look into a manger he had set up as a prop. I had intended to send him a copy of this. I don't know if I ever did. (That is one of the unfortunate side effects of brain surgery.) After you have read it, will you please pass this on to Father Dan with gratitude for his suggestion?

With love and prayers,

SURRENDER

Mimi wrote this note of encouragement to Melody, her Chinese friend sometime after she spoke to the group.

April 23 evening

Dear Melody,

I want you to know that I will be walking this weekend (April 24–25) in the American Cancer Society's RELAY FOR LIFE. At nine o'clock Saturday evening, I have requested that a luminary (lantern) be lit in honor of your courageous fight as a cancer survivor.

I hear from Chiu-yee that you are feeling weak and chilled. I send out the love and warmth in my heart to you. I am sorry you are uncomfortable. I am also sorry that you are feeling weak because I know that makes you sad. You want to give so much to your family, but you are not able to do what you wish. That is frustrating, I know. I am sorry for your frustration.

Chiu-yee tells me that you are having difficulty sleeping. I know how hard it is to lie awake at night and alone as fears and anxieties creep into our minds. My prayer for you is that you will continue to surrender your life to GOD. Rest quietly at night in His strong and loving arms. I know He cares for you so much and loves you more than we can imagine. I know this because He created you and made you the special person you are. He gave you a loving family and shaped you into the lovely, gentle woman you are. God has surely blessed you with Homer who works so hard and is strong for his family. God created within you those two wonderful sons, Kevin and Kendon, and God gave them intelligence and wisdom so they would be a special treasure to you.

I know your family is proud of you. We are all very proud of you. You have suffered through your cancer with dignity and grace, and you continue to do so. I want so much for your pain to end, but I also wish for you the comfort and strength to continue to live fully if this is God's will.

We all must surrender to God's will and I pray that He will send you comfort and that He will send your family a sense of peace, understanding, and acceptance. If you continue to live each day knowing that God is smiling upon your courage and Loving you more for your tremendous effort, I believe you will find comfort and peace.

This is my wish for you, dear friend. Although I have only known you for a short time, I feel very close to you because we have shared some of the same heartache of a cancer diagnosis. I do believe that each of us, through our disease, has grown stronger in our faith. In this growth of Christian maturity, we have taught our children much. We have grown to love our family and friends more deeply. We've continued to be good daughters, wives, mothers, and friends. Whether it is God's will that we live on earth or in Heaven with Him, we have made a difference in many people's lives and will continue always to influence those we love.

I will be out of town from April 27 to May 2. I hope to see you when I return. I keep you and your family in my thoughts and prayers always.

CHAPTER 6

Pat

I had been introduced to Mimi and had talked to her a few times after I was first diagnosed with breast cancer, but I did not get to know her and become friends until my breast cancer had metastasized to my lymph nodes. We scheduled our chemo on the same day so we could visit. We had many months of chemo together, but I will never forget those first few weeks. The fear you go through when you have a reoccurrence of cancer is ten times that of your first diagnosis.

Mimi's positive attitude and encouragement was just what I needed. Just being around her brightened everyone's day. She gave me a book to read *Facing Cancer with God's Help* and would have me read different verses from the Bible. This helped a lot. We also shared stories of our families, trips we were taking, side effects from chemo and radiation treatments, and life in general. Our ability to laugh and enjoy life through its many hardships is what got me through to remission.

Mimi's strength, courage, and love of God and humanity until the very end will always be with me and help me through whatever lies ahead.

Nancy Pelton
Friend and fellow cancer patient

May 1997

IN HIS TIME

This next series of writings are concerning Mimi's friend Pat.
Pat was a fellow cancer patient.
This is a letter of encouragement that Mimi wrote to her.

May 28, 1997

Dear Patty,

Since I spoke to you this morning, I have been busy speaking with my friends from church. Don't worry , Patty, we've got you covered . . .

I asked the entire congregation to pray for you, as we bring special petitions to God daily. This loving group of people has prayed for me daily since I was diagnosed with cancer. Now they also pray especially for you. Some shared their thoughts with me and offered me Bible verses that I think will comfort your weakened and frightened Spirit.

In addition, Monsignor's homily focused on Geese as they fly in V-formation. I looked for something in his homily to bring to you . . . and I found it. In the V-formation, the final duck is able to use much less energy as the troop flies through the air. The lead ducks take the brunt of the wind resistance, allowing other ducks at the back of the pack to rest against the currents of life. Pat, you've got to lay back and be that final bird for a while now. God is the lead goose! Your family, doctors, nurses, friends, prayer partners, and work cohorts are all flying for you to protect you and give you rest. Forget "Trying to be Strong" for others. Others can be strong for you. Allow them to be "for it is in giving that we receive." You will find in your family, as I did in mine, that their capacity to give runs deeper than we could imagine. We just have never wanted to test them, but God calls the plays here and not us. Giving can make all of them stronger, and you will become stronger as your love and appreciation for each of them grows. The big concept here is SURRENDER. SURRENDER your life temporarily to the care of others AND SURRENDER TO GOD. After all, He's been in charge here for a long time. He knows how to arrange things better than we do . . .

My friend, Amparo, suggested I share this verse with you:

Paul, in the Bible, was given many physical hardships in his life, YET through them he learned to trust and depend on God. 2 Corinthians 12:7–10 says,

"To keep me from becoming conceited because of these surpassingly great revelations, there was given me a thorn in my flesh, a messenger of Satan, to torment me. Three times I pleaded with the Lord to take it away from me. But he said to me, "My grace is sufficient for you, for my power is made perfect in weakness." Therefore I will boast all the more gladly about my weaknesses, so that Christ's power may rest on me. 1That is why, for Christ's sake, I delight in weaknesses, in insults, in hardships, in persecutions, in difficulties. For when I am weak, then I am strong."

Another verse that I have grown to love is this one:

Do not let your hearts be troubled.
Trust in God trust also in Me.
In My father's house are many rooms;
if it were not so, I would have told you.
I am going there to prepare a place for you,
And if I go and prepare a place for you,
I will come back and take you to be with me
That you also may be where I am.
You know the way to the place where I am going.

To me this declares God's love for all his people. He has a mansion in Heaven, and He is preparing a room for each of us. My room is not ready yet. Pat, I don't think yours is either. No one knows for sure when their room will be ready, but we need not fear because we know that when we do arrive, God will reside there with us. The way to the mansion is to live a good life and to offer all of our sufferings, insecurities, and disappointments for the greater Glory of God. When we do this we ARE LIVING EACH DAY TO THE FULL.

I always add my personal request to God's invitation to His Mansion. I tell God that I'm just not ready yet. He understands, and He likes when you talk to Him nicely. I acknowledge that He knows best, but He is never put off by my requests and He honors them. He has a history of listening to requests from his people. This prayer from good King Hezekiah in ancient times is recorded in the Bible, and I was especially moved by it when I read it:

Hezekiah was dying of a then incurable disease. He shed many tears. (He was a macho king so that means it's certainly all right for us to do the same thing.) He begged God to let him live. God said,

"Then the word of the LORD came to Isaiah: "Go and tell Hezekiah, 'This is what the LORD , the God of your father David, says: I have heard your prayer and seen your tears; I will add fifteen years to your life. And I will deliver you and this city from the hand of the king of Assyria. I will defend this city."
Isaiah 38:4–6

Our God is the same God yesterday, today, and for always, so I figure He will do the same for me and for you, if it be His will.
Hezekiah then gave thanks for his illness and recovery:

But what can I say?
He has spoken to me, and he himself has done this.
I will walk humbly all my years
because of this anguish of my soul.
Lord, by such things men live;
and my spirit finds life in them too.
You restored me to health
and let me live.
Surely it was for my benefit
that I suffered such anguish.
In your love you kept me
from the pit of destruction;
you have put all my sins
behind your back.
Isaiah 38:15–17

All of us should realize this every day of our lives.
Patty, I know God is with you and I pray that He will caress you as you undergo your surgery and recovery. I pray that he will fill the doctors' minds with His Almighty Wisdom and that He will be the Guide as He works through the doctors' hands.
God has been in control since your beginnings, and we ask Him to protect you now,

O LORD , you have searched me
and you know me.

You know when I sit and when I rise;
you perceive my thoughts from afar.
You discern my going out and my lying down;
you are familiar with all my ways.
Before a word is on my tongue
you know it completely, O LORD .

You hem me in-behind and before;
you have laid your hand upon me.
Such knowledge is too wonderful for me,
too lofty for me to attain.

Where can I go from your Spirit?
Where can I flee from your presence?
If I go up to the heavens, you are there;
if I make my bed in the depths, you are there.
If I rise on the wings of the dawn,
if I settle on the far side of the sea,
even there your hand will guide me,
your right hand will hold me fast.

If I say, "Surely the darkness will hide me
and the light become night around me,"
even the darkness will not be dark to you;
the night will shine like the day,
for darkness is as light to you.

For you created my inmost being;
you knit me together in my mother's womb.
I praise you because I am fearfully and wonderfully made;
your works are wonderful,
I know that full well.
My frame was not hidden from you
when I was made in the secret place.
When I was woven together in the depths of the earth,
your eyes saw my unformed body.
All the days ordained for me
were written in your book
before one of them came to be.

How precious to me are your thoughts, O God!

How vast is the sum of them!
Were I to count them,
they would outnumber the grains of sand.
When I awake,
I am still with you.
Psalm 139: 1–18

My friend shared this prayer, in time of ordeal, with me this afternoon so I could share it with you. It is all of Psalm 86 and it's a good one.

Hear, O LORD , and answer me,
for I am poor and needy.
Guard my life, for I am devoted to you.
You are my God; save your servant
who trusts in you.
Have mercy on me, O Lord,
for I call to you all day long.
Bring joy to your servant,
for to you, O Lord,
I lift up my soul.

You are forgiving and good, O Lord,
abounding in love to all who call to you.
Hear my prayer, O LORD ;
listen to my cry for mercy.
In the day of my trouble I will call to you,
for you will answer me.

Among the gods there is none like you, O Lord;
no deeds can compare with yours.
All the nations you have made
will come and worship before you, O Lord;
they will bring glory to your name.
For you are great and do marvelous deeds;
you alone are God.

Teach me your way, O LORD ,
and I will walk in your truth;
give me an undivided heart,
that I may fear your name.

I will praise you, O Lord my God, with all my heart;
I will glorify your name forever.
For great is your love toward me;
you have delivered me from the depths of the grave.

The arrogant (cancer cells) are attacking me, O God;
a band of ruthless men seeks my life-
men without regard for you.
But you, O Lord, are a compassionate and gracious God,
slow to anger, abounding in love and faithfulness.
Turn to me and have mercy on me;
grant your strength to your servant
and save the son of your maidservant.
Give me a sign of your goodness,
that my enemies may see it and be put to shame,
for you, O LORD , have helped me and comforted me.

Patty, as always, my thoughts and prayers are with you. Fall asleep knowing that God holds you (the morphine button accentuates this), and know that we all love you. Think strong and happy thoughts . . . and help those good cells divide and conquer!

Aug 1997

PREPARING TO DIE

This is a reflection on a conversation Mimi had with Pat when Pat needed encouragement and help in facing death.

August 13

Today I slept 'til 11:00. It felt good—it's the first day I did that since I heard about Tony's office troubles . . . My nerves finally got some of the rest they needed. I felt stronger. Pat Duke called at—actually come to think of it her call woke me up at 11:08 A.M. She asked if I could come over for a visit. I said I'd be there at 12:30. Shelley was there and had brought over In N' Out Burgers. Shelley had to leave soon and go back to work. Jim went out for a haircut, and I stayed with Pat.

Partway into our conversation, she told me that she figured she would be "like this" for six weeks to six months. She has only been home from the hospital for a couple days. I figured she was saying that she needed about six weeks to six months to recover. She said no that is how long she has to live.

She is scared of being in a lot of pain. She has suffered so long (cancer returned with a vengeance on Jan. 1 of this year) and been warned so many times that she is not going to live. Dr. Dosier is terribly frank, but he considers it his duty to warn people so they can prepare for the trip. It sounds, this time, like Dr. Shambaugh and Dr. Davis concur on her prognosis. I don't know for sure. It sounds like she has nodal involvement and her liver has cancer.

Pat is trying to prepare herself for dying, but she says it is so hard to say good-bye to her family. They encourage her to get up and walk, to eat, to get out so she can build up her strength for the fight. They want her to go back to chemo. She considers the idea but hates to put up with the side effects. She would rather be coherent and feel relatively good if she only has a short time left on this earth.

She says she doesn't know how to talk to God eloquently. I told her He is not looking for eloquence but for sincerity. She says she can't talk of God and dying without crying—so she doesn't talk about Him easily. I told her that I used to be that way, but I have become bolder. I asked for the Spirit to help me. She, I assured her, can ask for that same Spirit . . .

We talked of the relationship of God, Jesus, and the Spirit. She says she cries every time she thinks of Jesus Crucifixion, but I told her that Jesus CHOSE to do it. He wanted to do it for His Father and for the people the Father loved so much but who sinned and turned their backs on God. So Jesus offered to become man and teach the people by His example how they should live. I said that when Jesus died, He promised a Spirit, and Advocate, a Counselor would come to them and reside in them forever, and this Spirit would explain to them the things of God. This Spirit would intercede for them to the Father.

Pat worries that she is not worthy of God's concern. I assured her that God considers her worthy of His love and of His care. He will be with her and walk with her through the remainder of this journey through life. God alone will determine how long the journey will last, and when it does end, weeks or months or even years from now, God Himself will pick her up in His arms and take her into His kingdom.

Pat has been overwhelmed, I think, by the seeming suddenness of the increasing severity of her prognosis and the pain of her most recent hospitalization. She was visited by Donna from Hoffman Hospice, and Pat asked Donna to refrain from coming for the time being. Pat needs time to process her feelings. Donna understands, but wants Pat to feel the security that Hospice care is there if and when Pat or her family needs it. Hospice care is not only for the well-being of the patient, but for a family in crisis who also needs some help in moving through difficult times. I know those people involved with Hoffman Hospice, and I love and trust them. They are the ones I would have chosen to walk with me through my final days. They are kind, compassionate, and most of all, they love and serve God.

Three years ago, my husband and my daughter prepared themselves to help me die. I thank God that He chose to let me live. I look to each day for the reason I live. Today one reason became clear. God sent me to Pat, and I will be part of her life. If necessary, I will be part of her death. I believe this is what God has chosen for me to do, and I will do it with pride, with confidence, with humility, and with the same LOVE I would show to a family member . . . for Pat and I and her family are bound together as brothers and sisters in the body of Christ.

Jesus said ,"Love one another as I have loved you." I will try my best to do that. I will love Pat as Jesus has loved me, and I know that is incredibly more than I, or any of us, ever deserved.

Oct. 1997

VICTORY

When Pat died in 1997, Mimi wrote this poem for her.
It is the same poem that her family used on her funeral program.

What do you do when the agony is too much to bear?
Seek God's Face and learn to love Him more.
He asks no longer that you be his hands reaching out on this
earth to do His work.
He invites you now to lay rest your hands—
those hands which prayed and sought His work to do
those little girl's hands with which you once discovered the
world around you,
the tender arms which held babies and directed little children in
the right way to live,
the working hands which kept a tidy house,
the fast flying fingers which typed so efficiently,
the loving hands which provided a ready reach
for those in need,
the tiny delicate hands which slip gently into the strong hands
of the man you love.
the weary hands that reach out and say to loved ones,
"I need you near."
Lay your hands to rest now, Pat . . . and seek the Face of God.
He loves you and you will see the love in His eyes.
You are His precious child.
He wants to take you to His heart, brave warrior.
Your battle is over.
YOU HAVE WON

Nov. 1997

SECRETARY TO SAINT

Mimi was also asked to speak at Pat's funeral. This is what she said. It is included here to show how Mimi touched so many people's lives and was able to understand what they were going through and offer them support.

I was sitting in my den early this morning thinking about Pat and what extra thing I could add to what I had already prepared to say about her this morning. I wanted something that was uniquely Patty, and then it occurred to me what I could say—I want you all to take a minute here and turn to the person next to you, whether you know them or not, and just say to them, "You are special. Thank you." And really mean what you say.

That is what Pat would have said to all of you if she were able to. I have seen her say that to otherwise unnoticed people. If there is one good thing that comes from having a disease like cancer it is that we can learn to say things like that to people.

I probably have not had the honor of knowing Pat as long as most of you. I came to know her in the past year and a half, the most difficult part of her life. I admired the humility and the grace with which she lived and sympathized with the confusion of being diagnosed with a disease as puzzling and as difficult to treat as cancer. We both suffered with the same disease, but we encouraged one another through fears and treatments.

I was sad to hear, last month, that Pat had decided to discontinue chemotherapy, but I understood that she had fought cancer long and hard and had given it all she had. I cried for her then and for all the people who have to make this decision. I called her at home a few times after that, but she was too weak and too sick to speak. I knew I would probably not see her again so I sat down and wrote this memory.

Pat never was able to read it, but Jim sat by her that day and read it to her. I know she heard it and I know she understood.

These are my memories about a very special soul friend:

Pat was a darling, little, blonde with spirit and a smile, and I liked her immediately that day we met outside the chemotherapy office. We talked for two hours and laughed about the inconveniences that cancer had caused in our lives.

I confessed then that I worked out some of my frustrations by scribbling my feelings down in my diary when I was upset. When I was in a more upbeat frame of mind, I would write my feelings down then too. Someday, I told Pat I hoped that I would be able to destroy the negative recollections and publish the positive ones. I confessed that this would take some doing, however, since I didn't type very well. In her typical thoughtful way, Pat told me that she was a good typist, and she would be happy to help me with my work.

So I began to share, with my new friend, the role that God played in helping me conquer my fears and cope with my disease. Pat was a marvelous encourager, and I like to think that both of us became closer to recognizing that God was there even in the trials of our lives. She once "commissioned" a young boy whose mother worked at Dole to copy a Ziggy comic strip. She wanted it even brighter and bigger than the artist himself had sketched it. Pat then took young Jesse's drawing, had it framed, and gave it to me to have as a reminder that everyday there was at least one good thing to be thankful for.

Pat knew the power of God in the world, but not too long ago, she confided that she was afraid God failed to notice her. I knew that wasn't true—for God has promised that He will be with each of us ALWAYS. In the final months of her life, I know she turned to God to help her through her crises. I invited her to my parish Church one day, where she was anointed by a childhood acquaintance of hers from Taft who is now a Monsignor. She sought out a church community and united her friends and family under that embrace of God's love. She chose to let God take control of her life as her cancer spread.

It is hard to say good-bye to the special friend I knew for too short a time. I guess now I will have to type my own book . . . for my friend has just been promoted from secretary to saint.

Nov. 1997

REFLECTIONS

After Mimi went to the funeral of her friend Pat, she sat down and wrote this to send to the family to give them comfort. That was just the type of person she was.

November 3, 1997

It's Monday and I'm sitting here trying to absorb the events and thoughts of this weekend. My friend Pat was buried, and I know, now, she is in a safe place, but I wish she were still here. I have learned so much more about her in the past two days. It is evident that I knew only saw a small slice of the person she really was, and I felt sad that I didn't get to know her longer. We all feel that way, I know.

My first clue as to the truly exceptional person she was came when I walked into the mortuary Friday evening alone. I had just read the newspaper obituary, which she had written for herself—I guess it comes naturally for a good secretary to do things like that, the last minute detail work. I blinked back tears when I saw my name mentioned as a special friend along with Paul and Nita. I couldn't believe I ranked up there with them in the final evaluation!

Well, I figured, if her close family and friends were there sitting by her at the mortuary, then I guessed I belonged there too. I didn't know what I would witness over there, but off I went. Now Pat had a stubborn streak, and she had stated, "simple casket, no flowers, no fuss." What I saw was a serene, lovely scene—a casket, beautiful flowers surrounding, and contemplative, quiet people, sitting conversing with one another in soft tones. The greeting I received by people I have only met once or twice was overwhelming, and oh, so incredibly warm . . . Jim and Nita hugged me into their family.

It was a special moment, and it affirmed for me the truth about the "pre-cancer" Pat whom I had never known. She was warm, fun, silly, sensitive, loving, caring, and welcoming—just as were those people whom she loved and with whom she chose to surround herself.

I don't mean just the family and friends who were there that night in the chapel, but all those who sent flowers when Pat had requested them not to, and all those who attended her memorial tribute. I realized that people just couldn't help but to honor her that way—I think some of them even had fun going against her wishes because, for once, she was powerless to stop them. The pastel, spring colors of so many of the blooms celebrated her sunshine personality and her gentle femininity. She might have roared like a lion when she had too, but she had the heart of a lamb. People were sad to see her gone away so soon. That's what those flowers said.

The simple casket she requested was replaced by a stunning one, the final gift of the strong man who protected this gentle woman. I thought of what Jim had said to me just a few days earlier, "Mimi, this is the hardest thing I have ever done. Nothing in our society prepares us for death and saying good-bye." Well, I know a leader can rise when he must and Jim, you rank in my mind as one of the great leaders. You may not have had a map to follow, but the road you took us all down in recent weeks was paved in pure love. You not only showed us how to say good-bye, but you welcomed all Pat's family, co-workers, and friends to celebrate the wonderful attributes of Pat, which will continue to develop in each of us as we think about her life.

Shelley and Christen, I see so much of Pat in each of you. Your looks, your charm, your quiet sensitivity, and your zest for life. I especially had to smile, Shelley, when you talked about your mom and how she told you that "you had to be nice to people." It didn't matter if you liked them or not. You still had to be nice and smile at them. I can so see Pat saying that to you little kids . . . and to you big kids now. She was a determined mom (you may have even thought her to be bossy sometimes), but even in the short time I knew her, I know that she "bossed" about the right things. She was a great lady. Her pride in you and those grandkids knew no bounds. Remember what I told you on Saturday—look for her in signs in things around you, in "chance" events that seem to just happen. I know better than to think that Patti just sits idle in eternal life—I'm sure she's still arranging things now in Heaven, and some of her little charms will find their way down here to you and the rest of us.

Nita and Paul, you are great friends, and I'm so glad I got to meet you through Pat. You are caring and giving, and I know you make the world a better place. I'd call your celebration of Pat's life a type of a surprise party you threw for your best friend, but I don't think Pat would have been surprised that you would do such a thoughtful thing. Nita, I loved your personal recollections at her memorial service. You two must have had some wonderful times together, and you all also learned to smooth over rough edges when necessary. I can envision Pat jumping on you at a former time in your lives when she felt "you were overextending your boundaries." She probably would have said that you were fussing too much on her behalf as she became more ill, and she would have said she didn't want you getting all carried away at her memorial celebrations—but sometimes we just have to do what we have to do! You displayed your Class . . . and hers. Thank you. You are beautiful.

Nancy and Brenda, yours was a truly heartfelt and loving farewell to your dear sister. Doug did a very fitting job at expressing your sentiments. Thank you for sharing with us the part of Pat's early life that we never knew. She was a diamond—tough but sparkly. She knew how to be both, and she came about it at such an early age. I think she continued to worry about her baby sisters even in her adult life. The cruel irony is that the tables turned when she became ill, and I could see she reached to Brenda's model of faith, took some of that wealth for herself, and shared it as best she was able with you, Nancy. Pat was always a great equalizer, a Robin Hood of sorts. She wanted everybody happy.

I was touched by the memories of Pat's bosses at Tenneco and Dole. I was humbled to have shared a podium with them, but then that is the way Pat would have conducted business. EVERYBODY has something special; rank was unimportant in the grand scheme of things. I found it especially touching that her former bosses and pallbearers at the gravesite removed their boutonnieres and wove them gently into the flower spray adorning her casket. These leaders honored the faithful woman who helped them be successful, the relative who graced their family celebrations, and the friend who truly deserved flowers.

The celebration of Pat's life was a very moving, touching, honest communion of all the people whose lives had been influenced in some way by this very special lady. It delighted my heart to have the minister of Pat's own home church present to conduct her memorial service. Thank you for honoring me by letting me share this time with you.

July 1999

IN MY THOUGHTS

*Mimi ran into Pat's husband sometime after Patty died, and she
wrote this letter to him later. It can give us all encouragement
if we are mourning the loss of a loved one.*

July 25, 1999

Dear Jim,

It was so good to see you last week at the gas station. As I said
then, "it was just meant to be." I had been thinking a lot of you lately—
and there you appeared. God has a way of placing people where He
wants them.

Jim, you remain in my thoughts and prayers. The publication of
the enclosed book, *Encouraging Hands, Encouraging Hearts* in late May
of this year caused me to remember Pat more acutely than usual. It
seems ironic that Patty was the one who had originally offered to help
me type my story . . . and SHE then is the one whom my first published
piece is honoring. She was a true gem, and there are so many times I
wish she were here to share an experience or a thought with. I am sorry,
Jim, I know the loss is so incredibly great for you. My loss is transient;
yours is all the time. I only knew her for a short time in brief periods
of interaction. You loved her, devoted your life to her happiness, and
planned to spend forever with her. It is so sad when true love must say
good-bye. I'm sorry for you.

I'm sorry you have had such a difficult time with loneliness and
depression, but it sounds like you are doing a commendable job in trying to beat the blues. One must do what he has to in times of grief
like this—getting away from the memories of the house, visiting with
friends, and going back to see your family sound like suitable ways
of trying to accomplish this. I hope in time that you will be able more
comfortably to be in your and Patty's home . . . and find true solace
there. I will pray that this will happen for you, and if Pat hears me, I ask
her to sprinkle some of her stardust down here to make you stronger.

I'm sorry this letter is delayed. I had intended to get it off right
away to you, but I have been dealing with a few side effects of chemotherapy and trying to make plans to get away for a couple weeks in

August. Perhaps after I return, we can schedule a lunch date . . . and celebrate Patty's life.

It was interesting that the week I met you at the Chevron station is the very same week that my little neighborhood Bible Study was studying the book of Job. While the book of Job is pretty heavy, I see that much of it parallels your life in recent years. You lost the woman you loved, your health, some of your income, and cash assets. That is a lot to deal with.

I know God may seem far away, but I need to remind you that God will never turn his back on you. If He seems far away, perhaps you have turned away in your pain. "Cast your cares upon Him because He cares for you." Our God is a patient God . . . and He will wait for your timing, just let Him know that you are trying. I know you are. My prayers are with you as you struggle to put your life back in order.

In addition to the book (Pat's story is on page 150–152), I also enclose a couple of the Psalms, which we studied along with the book of Job . . . and they brought comfort to me. I hope they will minister to you as well.

Jim, please give my kindest regards to Paul and Nita, and to your loving family, especially Joy.

You remain in my thoughts and prayers.

CHAPTER 7

Perspective

Awhile ago, Liz called me and asked if I could write something about Mimi. After thinking about what our frienship was and what it meant to me, I said yes.

I met Mimi at our dental office. We became very close friends and had wonderful, joyful times full of laughter and deep thoughts. I will never forget when I came to bring her a gift on her birthday the first year I knew her. She celebrated it and she was so gracious. Then she said, "Amparo, you are my best friend!"

Liz responded, "Of course, she is your only friend." I decided then to share with her all the wonderful friends I had. Pretty soon, she was very popular, and I always rejoiced at the love everyone had for her.

After two or three years, she had extensive back reconstructive surgery. I thought this was hard for anyone. She was calm and always with a smile, which was her signature, one of the many gifts God had given her. Then on the year of her 46th birthday, she told me about this pain in her back. By the time her birthday came, she was diagnosed with colon cancer. This was hard to believe and hard to take.

All throughout, Mimi kept this same beautiful smile and loving way towards everyone. Mimi enjoyed life. This strength was a manifestation of her faith and her relationship with the Lord. Everyday she could, she would attend mass. Even when she had brain surgery, she was smiling. She battled cancer the same way.

I was diagnosed with Valley Fever recently. I have been very sick. So I'll do as Mimi would tell me. I'll live my life as she led hers. Mimi is still very close to my heart. I give thanks to God for the gift of Mimi during part of my life.

Amparo Kinnsch
Friend and prayer partner

1996

EXPRESSING GRIEF

*Mimi understood the importance of expressing grief but also that every-
one expressed grief differently. This is her perspective on grief.*

One of the things I have come to learn and appreciate is that you
must be open and try not to take offense at different people's responses
to a critical situation. I have seen the gamut of how people handle grief.
I was eight when my grampa died, and I slept in my grandmother's
room afterwards so she would have someone to "be there" in the dark
lonely night. She woke up every night just sobbing and talking to Pa
and telling him how much she missed him. I couldn't experience her
pain, but I could feel how much she loved him. I felt sorry for her, but I
felt happy for Pa. It was nice to be loved that much. My other Grampa
died when I was 15, and that Gramma and all her family were very
respectful and very stoic about the entire event. He was buried with
dignity, and that pretty much was the end of that.

One of my classmates died during our senior year of high school
after a two-year struggle with bone cancer. Peggy was brilliant, one of
ten children in a very close knit family. Her mom was with her the
night she died and recalled to us Peggy's parting words, "Mom, please
don't cry for me . . . if you could only see the vision that I see right now,
you couldn't possibly be sad." Peg was waked in her own living room
because that was her request. She said this part of her life should be
spent where she had her happiest memories. That taught me that dying
was a natural part of life, just a more sacred, solemn ceremony.

When Tony was in his medical residency program, a neighbor's
little boy was dying from a neuroblastoma. His parents were strong,
but he was stronger. When I went to visit one day, I was shocked at his
emaciated little body. The strange part is that he had no idea he had
cancer or that he was so emaciated-looking. He was behaving like any
other 3-year-old. His mother said there was no strength in his body
that should have allowed him to keep going the way he was. Problem
is: Nobody told Greggy that. Unfortunately, his steam ran out. He died
three days later, but my lasting reminder will always be that mind over
matter memory.

Before Tony's medical residency was over, we witnessed the
passing of another very close friend and cohort. His chief resident in

radiology, Pete, was diagnosed with leukemia. Since he received his treatments out of town at National Institutes of Health in Bethesda, Maryland, we other medical wives cared for his little boy so Pete and his wife Sheryl could have quality time together. Pete eventually died, and sadly, so did their little boy. I will never forget Sheryl's honesty and strength. She taught us how to walk gracefully with impending death, to accept it humbly, and move on with life. (She has moved on with life—that quality time with Pete left her with a beautiful little girl who was only a few months old when her daddy died. Heidi just turned 22, and she and her mom and step-dad have a very special relationship.)

Mary Martha Lazarus

May 2000

THE SURVIVOR'S RUT . . . AND HOW TO RISE ABOVE IT

Mimi was human just like the rest of us and got down from time to time.
Yet she was always able to gain perspective and rise above the bad.

We all get into a rut from time to time, and I was there, just scraping by. I just didn't realize it . . .

I was approaching my seventh year since being diagnosed with Stage 4 colon cancer. I had never been officially off chemotherapy except for brief periods when I had surgery, or when my blood counts were so low as to make chemotherapy do more harm than good, or occasionally when I went traveling for a week or two usually to a special family celebration, or to join my husband at an out of town meeting.

Each day was pretty much the same, mostly satisfying in a very quiet way. I was always recovering, it seemed, and so I acted that way. I slept late, took naps, and spent energy on fixing healthy meals. I went for chemotherapy and got recharged usually by the encouraging attitudes of the staff at the cancer center. I went to Mass daily and refocused on the goodness of God, networked with Spiritual friends, and felt the web of prayers that united us all. "Where two or three are gathered together in My name, there am I in the midst" gave me a reason to live.

I have always been a do-for-others type of person. Although there was not a whole lot I was able to do in a physically active capacity, I could pray with my mind and spirit. I could encourage through my words. I could get out and accomplish simple tasks with my somewhat burdened body . . .

I couldn't hold down a job; I had no kids at home anymore so the days were pretty quiet. I missed circulating. My computer was hardly a suitable daily companion, and the stories sleeping in my head were just that—they were sleeping! They did not possess the excitement or enthusiasm to create themselves a life on the page. Excuse me, I should be more honest. It was I who lacked the energy and enthusiasm to bring them alive upon the page.

Then I got hugged by a little girl, who looked at me, and assumed I was cured of my disease. Her trust convinced me that I was. For in her mind, I WAS fine. I could drive to the park, walk to the campsite, talk to the people, and help move the display into place. I could pick up a forty-pound child, pure love, and hug her to my chest. I could hold her baby sister, and bounce her through the air to make her laugh. I could walk the Survivors' lap of the Relay for Life, holding onto the hand of a friend who'd just been newly diagnosed, and I could laugh with friends as the day went on, and I could cry as I walked the lantern lap at the end of the day in the footsteps of my friends who no longer walked on earth. Of course, I was healed. I just didn't realize until a child told me.

Healed is a state of mind. Physically, I still have cancer. My body is still fighting a disease that can kill. Spiritually, I have always been and will always be alive—that was God's plan for me since the beginning of time. Mentally and emotionally, I'm as alive as I aim to be. That's what I had lost sight of.

Jan. 1998

HAPPY HOUR

This was written in the first part of 1998. It shows that even when Mimi had a bad attitude, it didn't last for long because she wouldn't let it.

Excuse me . . . but I was having an attitude problem.

Frequently we've heard cocktail hour referred to as "Attitude Adjustment" time. Young singles anticipate it, happy couples await it, business men participate in it, friends congregate in it, and bartenders concentrate in it. Everyone at times feels they need to let go of the stresses of life and seek relief at least temporarily.

What do cancer patients and happy hour participants have in common?

They both need an attitude adjustment sometimes.

I have decided that I have a very active imagination sometimes. I like that. In fact, I cultivate it. I feel good when it is active and alert, but sometimes it runs wild I dream of all the things I want to do, then feel disappointed when I can't accomplish them all.

I have a headache, surely my brain tumor is back. I am exhausted, and despite the fact that I have the flu and have had two chemos in that time, I'm sure my fatigue means that my liver is not functioning, and that's why I'm lethargic. My CEA is rising; surely that means the cancer is getting out of control

Four people I know have died this week alone (Helen Malerich, Mrs. Alexander, Rod Grimm, and Garlin Mixon.) I am sure no one gets out of this world alive . . . and I'm next.

A little bit of information can sometimes be a dangerous thing (CEA levels). I couldn't begin healing until I recognized there was a problem.

Fr. Davis sermon—growing up on farm. Crops grow well with cultivation and working of the soil. Hearts grow well with the same two things. When we allow our hearts to become hard, it is very difficult for the fruits of the Spirit to grow in them (Wed 1–28–98).

Christmas time—Giving my physical self—cook, clean, decorate, bake, launder. I gave of myself—my time, my energy, my concern. I wanted to reestablish the old me, the mom, the boss. I missed the opportunity to sit back, relax, visit with my adult children—and give to them the greatest gift of all—the God in me. He is not subject to exhaustion or depletion. His resources are endless. After all, He is God.

I have turned my life into an academic, mental analysis, and that has made me aware of perceived limitations of my brain (a sensitivity). I survived three years on Faith and Love. Then it took a vacation.

August—my mind was gearing toward getting off chemo after a year of "precautionary" treatment following adrenal mets. That was my program for happiness (see Beatitudes). I have not been very flexible. I have at least six worthy books I want to read. I had my goals list—yellow paper somewhere. I have insurance crabs and claims overdue. I have daily spiritual things I want to do. I have no energy. I have no discipline.

The good things. Tony listened to my feelings about chemotherapy (Jan. 22). He called Dr. Patel. Amparo listened, Irene listened, Mary Richard listened, Kathy Brown asked. Shirley Cove and Carolyn listened. My BSF fellowship asked. Mary Richard asked me to go to Heavenly Me. Judith let me help her. I ran into Michelle Mixon in the grocery store, found about Rick's dad, shared eulogy. Had coffee with Toni and Deb, got a sympathy card for John. Jackie Coppola sent a card today. I made time to let the Spirit in—while writing to John and Rick, shopping for cards for Judith to send girls, and sitting in the bathtub reading the Beatitudes. Ravi Patel left a message on the recorder, saying I'm stable (are you making that up or is this the placebo effect—trust him either way). Paul Czysz enthusiasm for brain project and empathy for my initial prognosis.

Focus-losing weight, healthy body. Now I have dimpled fat instead of plum fat. WOW!

Jeff Lane and Ingrid Olson

My mind was gearing toward getting off chemo and now I am working toward accepting that this is not the time. It takes energy to work toward this acceptance. For now I have to remain on it.

Corey: What does chemotherapy symbolize to you, for you?

Life. I know that is a main reason I'm alive . . . but I worry that it is having long range effects on my body.

Early 1996

LIVE

Mimi wrote this during her first year of cancer treatment. She thought first of other people not of herself. It shows of her reaction to the diagnosis of cancer.

CANCER? CANCER! CANCER. How am I supposed to respond?

How do I tell my mother over the phone? How can my husband with tears in his eyes be happy again? How can I reassure my children who are trying so hard to be strong?

They all think people die of cancer. Some do. I'm not. I won't die with cancer. I will choose to LIVE with cancer . . . until my time is over. I don't know how long that will be. Nobody does.

I will live each day as if there is no tomorrow and hope that it will last forever. Right now I will live one day at a time. It reminds me of that line from Shakespeare, "We are but players on the stage who strut and . . ."

That is what we all are about. Our birth brings us into the drama. We arrive, we play out our part, and carry on through the continuum until we cease to play, and make our exit from this world. That's the same ending for all of us.

While we are here, life can be truly beautiful . . . if we put our heart and soul and spirit into it. Time is valuable. Use it well. Life is precious.

Relationships are important. God makes it meaningful.

March 2001

THE BONUSES

These are Mimi's reflections after finishing radiation in 2001.
Ellie is the radiation nurse who Mimi befriended over the years.

March 30, 2001

Ellie: What will you do now that radiation is finished?

Mimi: I'll still be around. This building is sort of my home away from home.

Ellie: I guess you do consider it sort of like that. I know I do— it's my home   away from home . . . but I get paid for being here.

Mimi: Oh, I get special bonuses from being here too . . .

One big bonus is the chance at Life.

Appreciation for the dedication of the doctors. Having a husband and two daughters who've gone the rigors of med school and residency and on into medicine, I know the devotion required to keep at it. I'm thankful for the combination of intelligence, wisdom, curiosity, intensity, compassion and faith that keeps them persevering through the stress and demands of their profession.

There is also the honor of getting to know and be in close contact with the nurses, technicians, and other support staff who work extremely hard, but willingly sacrifice and share some of their personal lives so that mine may be more meaningful.

The patients, some of them stronger than me, some weaker than me, some younger, some older who make me cry . . . and want to fight harder. Or who make me smile and make me remember how vital it is to have a positive attitude.

1997

THE ROLLER COASTER RIDE

*This gives us insight into Mimi's perspective on cancer and
the subsequent treatments.*

Today as my mind is thinking toward an end of a three-year course of chemotherapy; I am feeling pretty positive. My oncologist asked how I am progressing on my book. He says he's not seen any rough drafts lately . . . and I apologized for my general lack of motivation these past six months. I feel it is not so much the cancer, which is getting me down, but other piddly things—physical, mental , and emotional that are either requiring an output of my energy or zapping the limited amount of strength I have.

The physical effects of chemotherapy have become pretty predictable. I can work with them. For example, on a weekly schedule I know I will feel bloated, nauseous, and generally irritable on the day of chemo. Antinausea medication will allow me to sleep through the night and well into day two. The worst effects will be gone by day three. It's like recovering from a short-lived flu bug where you feel wonderful to be over the crisis, but you have that just awakening from hibernation period when you are generally nonfunctional and unmotivated to do much of anything.

Once over that hump, there is a burst of energy, a desire to do something exciting, a need to organize or accomplish something useful. This mood lasts generally for another 30 hours or so, and then comes a period of fatigue for an afternoon or an evening. The fourth day usually brings a return of physical symptoms as the chemotherapy is working at the cellular level. Gastrointestinal distress, in my case, diarrhea commonly creeps up. It's not a good day to be out and about, unless readily available and accessible restrooms are close by.

Following this day, I have a two good days in which to accomplish a week's worth of activities because tomorrow the cycle begins again.

Life is what I call a roller coaster ride. Sit down, strap yourself in, realize you have little or no control over the situation. Be exhilarated by the highs. You laugh and scream and accomplish as much as you can. Then be scared by the lows. Worry what will happen next, withdraw, and wish the ride would end.

Early 2002

SPIRITUALITY AND HEALING

Mimi's philosophy on living with cancer served her well, here is some insight into what her philosophy was.

There are numerous studies currently showing that prayer/ spirituality plays a role in physical healing. We can choose to busy ourselves reading these scientific data collections of study, or we can choose to walk forward in faith and be a part of the living experience of such scientific revelations. Many will choose to gather all the facts first and decide for themselves if this is a credible conclusion; others will embrace the experiment while it is being conducted.

I prefer the experiential route. This one takes in all the human characteristics like curiosity, community, comradeship, and creativity. It requires preparation of both one's physical and mental attitudes, for it is an invitation to vulnerability because a sincere, seeking heart will have to trust that it or another human being possesses the spirituality to serve as a conduit for God. Do I trust enough to try it?

Mid-1997

FAMILY

Mimi reflects on her first few months with cancer.

Christine was a final year medical student. Being a doctor had been her goal since she was a young child. She had entered the final stretch and was working on the oncology service when she got word of my diagnosis. She knew the facts. Within a day she was home in Bakersfield on leave of absence from medical school. She was in effect prepared to temporarily suspend her life goals to come home and help me. She had come home to help me die. I didn't die. The devotion of my family and my friends gave me conviction to live, to fight back against the disease that threatened to destroy me.

Christine and her father were the only people in the family fully aware of how serious my diagnosis was. They bore a heavy burden.

She had come home to help me die. "How did that make you feel?" I was asked. Proud. "Proud, why?" Because we had raised a child who was willing to give up what was most important in her life to come home and help me. That care, that concern, that love made me want to remain her mother, to see her dreams fulfilled, to show her how attitude and appreciation for God's world could enhance the lives of everyone.

I was expected to live for two weeks to two months. I did not know that at the time of my diagnosis. I will always be grateful to my family and my doctors for never telling me so. That would have deprived me of my hope. I'm afraid that if I knew, I may have circled the due date on my calendar and lived up to that day, then died . . . as had been expected.

Early 2000

GOING WITHIN

Mimi began the practice of meditation during the course of her illness. This gives us her perspective on that art form.

In the depth of meditation, there are no fears or concerns, for the peace of God pervades. I have been graced with knowing these moments of God's peace through the kindness of instruction on the process of meditation, the practice of discipline for getting to that quiet place, the repeated effort of fighting off distracting thoughts, and the desire to surrender to God.

When I meditate, God meets me in my quiet place. We become one in Spirit, often only for a brief moment. I know God is there, and I am soothed with His peace. "Be still and know that I am God (Psalm 46:10). Throughout the day, God blesses me in ways and in places I don't expect. The peace that I experience in meditation comes back to me sometimes in troubled moments when I close my eyes and come to silence. Sometimes it comes to me immediately, ironically it is unlike those times when I sit for scheduled meditation sessions and end up vigorously fighting off the demons of distracting thoughts.

One of these moments when God's grace comes easily is when I lie in sterile radiology rooms on MRI or CT tables. I close my eyes and become perfectly still as the scanning procedures begin. I repeat my mantra to counteract the mechanical sounds of science—the banging, the whirring, the chirping sounds that go on within the tube. I cast off my fears and anxieties as the Peace of God transcends the trivial multiplication process of my cancer cells. I know I am beloved of God. He can caress my body, and He is fully aware of the nature of those cells within me, "For You knit me together in my mother's womb. I praise you because I am fearfully and wonderfully made (Psalm 139: 13,14)."

Often as I recover from the after effects of weekly chemotherapy, I am able to get into the Silence of God with ease. Perhaps the affects of the medication eliminate distraction. Maybe I am simply too exhausted to do anything or care about anything, but I know that the unconditional Love of God sustains me.

I will carry that Love as I move into the day and into the week, as my strength and energy level gradually improves. I will recall that Peace as I go out into the world. I have learned that with my illness,

I walk with God. We have been going through this trial together for almost six years. Tests, surgeries, chemotherapy, and recovery come in a seemingly never-ending cycle. When I become impatient with my human frailty or become frustrated by my changed lifestyle, I need to remember this is where God wants me now. I need to close my eyes more often and beckon Him to come. *Maranatha.*

Mimi Deeths
Bakersfield, California
March 2000

Early 1998

TRUST

Mimi's letters to others also give us great insight into how she dealt with her disease.

January 29

(I began this letter right after I spoke to you, then I had to have chemotherapy and did not get back to it for a week. I have thought about you and prayed for you everyday. That is one positive thing we can all do during recovery times-seek God for ourselves and pray for others.)

Dear Susan,

I am so happy you felt that you could talk to me today. I understand how frustrated you must be and how fearful you are about facing a reoccurrence of your cancer. Cancer is a mean disease, and even the strongest people have a hard time battling it. I personally don't know how any person on his or her own can deal with cancer, but I do know that any person with the help of God can overcome any trials, suffering, or uncertainty. God will help you as he has helped me, but we must go to him humbly and ASK HIM.

Don't forget God in your times of greatest need, Susan. HE IS THERE FOR YOU. He understands your distress. He understands your pain. God Himself became a man, Jesus, and that man-God felt everything that we feel. He felt the rejection of people. People denied the teachings of Jesus. People chased Jesus out of their towns. People turned against this perfect man who was without sin—and they crucified Him. Therefore, when we feel persecuted and when we suffer, Jesus understands our pain.

Cry to Him for help and for strength as He cried to His Father in the Garden of Gethsemane. Jesus was under tremendous stress, and asked his Father if it was possible to remove the cup He would willingly drink of. God the Father chose not to remove the suffering because He knew that by suffering Jesus would save all men from original sin. He saved me and He saved you. If You were the only person in the whole world who needed to be saved, Jesus would have died for you alone. HE LOVES YOU THAT MUCH!

February 5

Finally, I am getting back to finishing this letter. Susan, I could tell in the short time that I talked to you on the phone that you have Jesus in your heart. Sometimes we forget. I know I do. I pray that we will both remember more often.

At church yesterday, I heard a reflection that helped me very much to remind me of my faith. I hope it helps you too. The woman who did our communion service read this from the Bible; then the woman conducting the service shared this thought with us.

In this gospel passage, Jesus is hurrying to the side of a little girl who has died. Jesus may be in a hurry and there may be crowds all around, but what does Jesus do? He takes time for the woman . . . and he takes time for each of us.

The woman with the hemorrhage reaches out IN FAITH. She has TRUST that He will help her and stop her difficult physical condition. Do we have that kind of faith? Do we trust that Jesus will help us, cure us. It may not be an immediate cure. This poor woman suffered for twelve years, and she had spent everything she had! She consulted doctors. I'm sure she went through the prescribed treatments of the time (surgery, medicine, primitive chemical therapy) as we must do BUT SHE KEPT THE FAITH and Jesus noticed. Jesus noticed so much, in fact, that the woman needed only to touch the hem of HIS garment and Jesus felt it. Jesus felt some of His power going out to the woman. Can you imagine—energy flowed out of Jesus' body into that woman's body. Jesus energy can flow to us, too, if we have the FAITH to reach out to Him. Remember, when we reach out to Jesus, He feels it . . . and He will respond. He loves us so.

I pray, Susan, you will reach out to Jesus. He will help you. He will heal you in body, mind, and Spirit. Be assured that my prayers are with you.

Nov. 1997

THE POWER OF GOD

*This letter again gives us perspective into Mimi's
thoughts on living with cancer*

November 13,1997

Dear Lizzy,

I talked to Mary Lue several days ago and heard for the first time that you and I had more in common than we ever hoped to have. I'm sorry to hear about your breast cancer, and I'm sorry that I did not know about it sooner. I would have offered my prayers up with all the others, which I know are being offered for you. I will, however, begin immediately praying for your full recovery and for your peace of mind and comfort during the remainder of your chemotherapy.

I'm sorry, Liz, about the chemotherapy. I know that breast cancer with nodal involvement is about the most obnoxious chemo there is. I'm not sure which one you are on—Adriamycin, perhaps—but never mind—they are all rough. I was a little disappointed that you did not choose a red wig or something really racy—I'm just kidding! You have always had a very classy look—and you might as well keep up the illusion of being classy even when you feel like_____! (Fill in the blank.) I say openly sometimes that I can feel like sh—, and I figure that is okay for me because I was diagnosed with colon cancer and "sh—is a big focus when you are dealing with that part of the anatomy. I don't say it out loud very often, but I mutter it to myself sometimes when I am especially mad.

Anyway, enough for the foolishness. Down to business. I feel like I can lead you along in this process because I am a veteran of sorts. I have been on chemotherapy. Six weeks on—one week off—six weeks on—one week off, etc. for three years. I never get time off for good behavior. The only time I can escape the stuff is if the MRI's show another tumor, and then I get to go off long enough to have surgery and recover. You will believe when I say there were times I was happy to have surgery so I could go off chemo. I hate it that much. I'm sure you do too. It's a mean treatment.

Liz, I have to say, very seriously, it is the reason I am alive today, and in many ways the last three years of my life have been the most meaningful so far. I realize each day to be a gift, and there is very little that I take for granted anymore. When I was diagnosed, the doctors told Tony that I probably would live for two weeks, possibly two months. I did not know this at the time. Christine got a leave of absence from medical school to come home and be with me. She knew the prognosis. She and Tony decided to keep this knowledge from the other three kids, and they did not feel that I needed to deal with it either.

At the time of my diagnosis, I had a tumor in my large intestine four inches from the rectum. I went to surgery expecting to come out with a permanent colostomy. Incredibly, although eleven nodes were involved, none of them were on the lower end of the tumor, thus my rectum was spared and a colostomy was not needed. I was soaring high on this fact alone . . . so much so that for my forty-fifth birthday, three days later, I had a huge piece of chocolate cake and never even got sick! Better yet, this is when the medical personnel advised me not to eat it because I was on a total liquid diet at the time because the surgeon had to remove 15 inches of intestine. Honestly, I was so starving from the liquid that the cake tasted wonderful . . . and I didn't need that extra fifteen inches of colon to digest birthday cake!

At the time of my initial surgery, my liver was inoperable because of four large metastatic tumors embedded in it and scattered tumors all over the surface of my liver. Chemotherapy was begun two weeks after having 15 inches of colon removed. It was just to shrink the liver tumors and buy me some time. God had a different plan. Over an eight-month period on chemotherapy, he made most of the tumors disappear and then used a UCLA liver specialist to remove two small tumors that stubbornly refused to disappear. Two and a half years later, I have no sign of liver cancer. Likelihood of my survival at the time of diagnosis was 0 to 6%. Science statistics sometimes neglect to consider the Power of God. I don't . . . and you better not either.

One of my rules is that I don't ask God why I have to have cancer. I have it. Period. So I ask instead, "God, what do you want to teach me?" Every day I ask Him that. Every day He gives me some answer. On the particularly quiet days, when He does not seem to answer, I have come to realize that His silence is giving me an answer. "Be patient, " He says. It took me a long time to realize that is what He was saying. I guess that is one of the advantages of having cancer for a long time—pretty soon you actually do learn to be patient.

Patience teaches you a lot. You learn to listen more because you are unable to DO. I have gotten into contemplative prayer. Try it. You sort of start with Yoga breathing, but add a special dimension. With every breathe you take in, carry a sacred word to your soul. "Jesus" is a good word to start with. (He understands your pain.) Try to use the same word everyday (less distraction, better discipline at least for beginners). As you breathe out, breathe out all the distractions of your day, the fears, the anxieties, the frustration, the piddly stuff that comes in to clutter your mind.

You might use this technique already, but in case you haven't tried it , TRY IT—YOU'LL LIKE IT! Upon occasion, I have experienced the embrace of God, I have felt the "fluttering" of the Spirit, I have heard a Gospel phrase that brought me strength, and I have had great peace. It is a great opportunity for God to speak to you. Our challenge is to clear our minds long enough to let that happen. I'm not sure what to call the experience, but I do think it is close to what I would say is an out of body experience . . . and let's face it, when you are on chemo, it can be quite desirable to leave the body behind. Usually, I try to do this for about twenty to thirty minutes. Sometimes, I get five seconds of inspiration, sometimes more like five minutes (out of 1/2 hour of prayer). The rest of the time is pleasant and a means of discipline, and it's far better use of my time than some of the other stuff I do—like worry, watch TV, read something useless, pity party, etc.

I will try to keep in better touch with you as your treatments progress. I have just recently started to try to wean off chemotherapy. The extent of time I have been on it is beginning to take a toll on my body—muscles, joints, skin, fatigue . . . so my doctors are letting me do a trial of every other week chemo and see if I still remain free of rising CEA (cancer antigen) counts and metastatic tumors. My body is better able to recover between treatments. On this new every-other-week schedule, I only have four "down" days and then ten good ones as opposed to the regimen of every week when I just feel yuk most of the time. This weaning has been going on for four months, but it is still too early to assess whether it is keeping my cancer in check or not. Again, patience comes into play . . . and faith!

Liz, I hope you are able to enjoy the relatively good times in between chemo sessions. My advice is not to waste it worrying what tomorrow will bring but to trust God in these matters and know that He is in charge. He already knows the end result of your cancer experience. Before we were even born, He knew the number of our days. I've figured out that since He made us, He also has the right to decide when He will recall us . . . so I try not to bother my little brain about THE BIG TIMETABLE. Rather, I try to make each day count and cling to this promise of God, "I know the plans I have for you," declares the Lord, " plans to prosper you and not to harm you, plans to give you hope and a future" (Jeremiah 29:11). This passage is my gift to you today. Use it everyday. I take it literally. I have to believe that He will give me hope and a future.

I try to utilize everything available. I use prayer and gospel words. I use scientific medicine (obviously), and recently, I began to utilize psychotherapy. I began to see Corey, a psychologist, in July of this year. Corey is a cancer survivor who leads the cancer support group at my oncologist's office. I dropped out of it after a couple months because it was too depressing—too many people were dying and not coming back to lend much support! Anyway, I felt I needed some support during this process of weaning off chemotherapy since I fear cancer growing out of control again, so I see Corey privately every week or two. We just talk things out. I feel like I can tell him of my insecurities, but I don't want to bother my family with them.

It did occur to me that my family has problems of their own associated with having to deal with my disease, but we don't tend to discuss them. There is some fear there and a lot of avoidance, on my part especially. I did, however, ask Katie to accompany me to one of my sessions with Corey before she left for her second year med school in August. We used up a whole box of Kleenex and cleared the air after a three-year period where we each tried to "protect the other." Katie, incidentally, took a year off between college and medical school to come home and be with me.

Corey got her and me to talk about that year and what each of our perceptions of it was. I said I was proud of myself because I turned to God in my uncertainty. Katie confessed that she had a hard time handling that because she herself did not possess that depth of faith, and my confidence made her feel "unworthy." Katie had her fears too. Scientific knowledge told her I would probably die of my disease during that year she was home. She would have been in charge . . . and she confessed she did not know how she would handle it. She wanted guidance from her mother at that time, but her mother was off on a faith experience. Katie wanted to discuss our lives together and bring us to closure if it was necessary. I was into Jeremiah where God promised me hope and a future! We were not on the same wavelength, and that was painful to her. I was not aware that she was feeling so insecure.

So Corey asked Katie at this session, if that was so important to her, why she didn't try to broach the subject with me? Katie started to cry and she said, "I wanted to but my mom's faith was so important to her. She had HOPE . . . and no matter how bad I (Katie) might have felt, I could never take that hope away from her."

Then it was my turn to cry. This child, whom I had tried to protect all my life, had been hurt by my silence. Sometimes love hurts. Cancer is a family disease, as I'm sure you have discovered, Liz. We, who must go through the physical burdens of the disease, must also recognize that our family and friends go through the mental stress, the uncertainty, the anxiety, the mood swings, and the pain with us. I have learned that it is better to talk about our feelings so we don't leave those around us "tiptoeing so as not to rattle us." Once we have talked out the most pressing problem, we have to drop it and reestablish our relationships because that affirms the value of that other person in our lives. It also helps us to go on with our cancer as true survivors.

Hang in there, dear friend. I love you and wish I was there to give you a great big hug . . . because I do understand. You remain in my thoughts and prayers.

CHAPTER 8

Speeches

Every time I think about Mimi, in my mind there's a smiling angel sitting there and saying to my wife (and other cancer patients), "Be strong. If I can do it, you can do it too, and I'll be on your side . . ." Then with the greatest motherly love and strong will, she is driving a long way to see her children.

Since we lived in the same subdivision, I had the great honor to see her around often. She always said, especially after some terrible days of treatment, she treated everyday as her last; she lived accordingly and used every day very well. She tried to encourage as many cancer patients as possible, and she never forgot her most precious gifts from GOD—her children.

Homer Kuo
Friend and Melody's husband

Mimi was a constant source of inspiration and strength, not only for my mother, but for me a well. The way she relied on God and then used the strength God gave her to inspire and encourage other people really impacted me. I also remember the love she showed to my mother by just stopping by our home to say hello and check on my mom.

Kevin Kuo
Friend and Melody's son

Jan. 1999

WOMEN TO WOMEN SPEECH

In 1999, Mimi was asked to give her testimony and introduce the speaker at a local conference. Dr. Gonzales was Mimi's psychologist for many years.

A friend sent me a quotation last week. When it arrived, I needed it because I had been sort of carrying on with one of my own private little pity parties. These words provided a little reminder that I needed to put things into perspective.

Four and a half years ago I was diagnosed with colon cancer already metastatic to my lymph nodes and to multiple sites in my liver. The operating room surgeon was able to remove my colon tumor and resect my colon, but he determined during surgery that it was not feasible to remove the tumors from my liver. There were too many of them, and my liver was inoperable at that time. The plans I had for my life seemed shattered. There was no where I could turn . . . except to God. Over the past four and a half years, I have come to know His love, His grace, and His faithfulness.

In addition to my faith, I have been blessed with a very supportive family, wonderful caring friends, and an oncologist who told me he would do everything he could medically to help me live. He has never failed in his promise.

I, however, had no idea all that his medical treatment would entail . . . over the past four and a half years, this has included six cancer related surgeries, several months on continuous 24-hour drip chemotherapy delivered directly through a shunt to my liver, and approximately 200 weekly IV sessions of systemic chemotherapy. Recent scans show no tumors evident anywhere in my body. However, my CEA tumor marker for colon cancer is still elevated so I have yet to enter the remission phase.

As many of you may know, chemotherapy can be very effective, but it does not come without side effects. I feel good three to four days each week and my outlook is positive, but those other days of the week I'm recovering from chemo and tend to feel fatigued, nauseated, irritable, and obnoxious. My bed is then my favorite place to hide out. I feel frustrated because I feel I am accomplishing nothing. Then I begin to feel good . . . and start rushing around to do all the "important" things I dreamed of doing when I was in bed. I have discovered that dreaming is far easier than doing. I can end up feeling bad on my good days because I try to accomplish too many things.

One of the most difficult and persistent issues I have had to deal with is the long-term roller coaster ride of physical reactions, fatigue, and emotional swings. I have come to realize that I am not alone on that roller coaster. I have discovered excellent resources in helping you cope—one is our local Cancer Society. There are good books available, and I recommend Coping, a magazine for cancer survivors. Our speaker for the evening has been featured on the cover of this magazine, and his article inside is very informative and helpful. Over the years, I have learned to better use honesty and tact in communicating with family members, physicians, and friends . . . and have come to value these team members as partners in helping me conquer my cancer.

I can communicate to others that I get stressed by small things sometimes, and I become anxious as new symptoms arise, each new order for blood tests, and MRI and CT scans are ordered. Since this is such an important part of my life right now, I've tried to learn ways of dealing with the stress and anxiety. I have worked with relaxation and visualization, and I have tried these techniques with my children and with friends, occasionally. I have seen these exercises help others and realize how effective these techniques can be in many different situations. By no means are they useful only for people who are ill—but can provide a period of "attitude adjustment" for anybody, anytime. Patients, caregivers, and friends can all profit from these "time out" techniques.

I know you are all excited to learn more of what I am talking about, and I am happy to introduce to you Dr. Corey Gonzales who will teach us some of these visualization/relaxation techniques. Corey is a 12-year cancer survivor. He began studies for his Master's degree while he was still being treated for cancer and was awarded his Doctorate degree in Clinical Psychology from the California School of Professional Psychology in Los Angeles. It is the only private, accredited doctoral program for psychology in the state. Corey has a full-time clinical practice here in Bakersfield, facilitates a cancer support group for patients and their families, has been published in Coping Magazine, and is a valued speaker for both the Man to Man lecture series and our Woman to Woman informational evenings.

He is a positive example for all of us. I don't think he will be insulted if you fall asleep—that only means he has effectively encouraged relaxation. Welcome him now, please, and then sit back, relax, and mellow out with Dr. Corey Gonzales . . .

Jan. 1999

SHIELDING LOVE

*When someone touched Mimi's life, she usually had to write a
thank-you letter to them to let them know. This was after
the Woman to Woman talk when she introduced the speaker.*

January 21, 1999

Dear Corey,

Thank you very much for speaking at our Woman to Woman group last Tuesday. I was really happy with the attendance and the response to the relaxation/visualization exercises. I'm glad you got it on tape. I hope it turned out well. It was nice to meet Jamie, and I'm so glad she came for the evening.

I thought your guided relaxation was superb. You know how I have certain "buzz" words . . .

You mentioned "a shield surrounding you." You repeated the word shield several times . . .

Well, two weeks ago in Bible Study we were studying Genesis 15 where God promises Abram, "I am your **shield.**" We studied this reference and looked up other references to God as our shield. I got so turned on about the references that I came home two weeks ago, looked them up and typed them up, made a bunch of copies, and mailed them to about twenty people whom I know are in need of this security. That made me happy . . .

Then Tuesday night you mentioned SHIELD again. It was like an unexpected affirmation and another sign that God is with us in all facets of our life—cool, huh?

I got some good news at chemotherapy yesterday. My CEA has dropped for the first time in eighteen months. It has slowly and steadily climbed since August of '97 (one to five points each month). Last month it dropped by five!!! From 38 to 33 . . . now if I can just keep that up . . .

Have a good couple weeks. Thanks to Jamie. I'll see you sometime in early February.

P.S. Enclosed is the shield sheet which I sent to my children, family members, and friends.

THE LORD IS MY SHIELD

This is the list Mimi made reference to in the last letter.

But you are a **shield** around me, Oh Lord;
You bestow glory on me and lift up my head.
To the Lord I cry aloud and He answers me from His holy hill.
I lie down and sleep;
I wake again because the Lord sustains me.
Psalm 3: 3–5

For surely, O Lord, You bless the righteous:
You surround them with Your favor as with a **shield.**
Psalm 5:12

Praise be to the Lord for He has heard my cry for mercy.
The Lord is my strength and my **shield.**
My heart trusts in Him and I am helped.
My heart leaps for joy,
and I will give thanks to Him in song.
Psalm 28:6–7

We wait in hope for the Lord Who is our help and our **shield.**
In him our hearts rejoice for we trust in His Holy Name.
May Your unfailing love rest upon us, Oh Lord,
even as we put our hope in You.
Psalm 33:20–22

He who dwells in the shelter of the Most High
will rest in the shadow of the Almighty.
I will say of the Lord, "He is my refuge and my fortress,
My God, in whom I trust."
Surely He will save you from the fowler's snare
and from the deadly pestilence.
He will cover you with His feathers,
and under His wings you will find refuge;
His faithfulness will be your **shield** and your rampart.
You will not fear the terror of the night,

nor the arrow that flies by day,
nor the pestilence that stalks in the darkness,
nor the plague that destroys at midday.
Psalm 91: 1–6

You are my refuge and my **shield;**
I have put my hope in Your Word.
Psalm 119:114

Do not be afraid, Abram,
I am your **shield**, your very great reward.
Genesis 15:1

ME?

These are thoughts that Mimi wrote in her journal after being asked to speak at a Hoffman Hospice event.

When you were born, you cried and the world rejoiced. Live your life in such a manner that when you die, the world cries and you rejoice.

Indian Proverb

1/25/96

I have recently become involved with Hoffman Hospice. My original connection is through Celestial Correspondence volunteer program. The role of a C.C. is to keep in touch weekly (through notes, cards, letters, phone calls) with a hospice patient or bereaved member of a patient's family.

When I was sick, I know how much a friendly greeting lifted my spirits. Grief over a lost loved one is similar to physical illness. It is always nice to know that someone cares. I have come to appreciate the value of a cheerful note and now I enjoy thinking each week that perhaps I can be successful in turning someone's ordinary day into a special occasion for a moment. My current correspondents are two teenage girls from two different families, each of whom has recently lost a parent or grandparent to cancer. I can sympathize with these young women, and it makes me feel good to be able to encourage them.

The coordinator, Rick, says I'm a good volunteer and recently asked if I would be willing to serve in a more active capacity. I told him I was hesitant because of my own current ongoing status with chemotherapy and unpredictable side effects. He asked if I might be interested in "special projects." I explained that I've always been a special projects person, and I'm good at licking stamps and stuffing envelopes at home in my free time. He laughed and said he would put a star by my name. "But really," he said, "I thought you'd be a good person to present a seminar for doctors and nurses. Do you think you might be interested in that?"

This question took me by surprise. I mumbled something about my poor public speaking ability to which Rick countered, "Well, could you maybe lip synch for us then?" I sensed Rick was not going to give up easily. So I bounced this idea off three people whose opinions I value—my husband, my close friend, and a nurse friend who is in my Bible discussion group.

My husband immediately answered. "I think that could be very gratifying. You should try it."

My close friend said, "You would be good. You are articulate. You've had experience and would have good advice to give. You should do it."

With my nurse friend, I explained the situation and told her I would feel insecure addressing nurses and would feel even more petrified addressing doctors. She asked, "Why? You're married to a doctor!"

Well, yes, I am married to a doctor and many of my social contacts are doctors. I have spoken at length with some of them about my medical problems and my feelings, and they listened. I guessed maybe other doctors would be attentive too. In addition, I think I have developed an easy, honest relationship with my own physicians . . . so what would be so scary about speaking to a group of physicians? The answer is the GROUP. Groups scare me. I felt a bond here with Moses in the Old Testament. Remember when God, in the form of a burning bush, appeared to Moses, and God told him that he wanted Moses to lead the Israelites out of Egypt into the Promised Land.

Moses' response to this request was "Who am I to go to Pharaoh, and lead all these people out of Egypt?"

God's thoughtful answer (Exodus 3: 13–14) was simply, "I AM has sent me to you!"

Well, it's hard not to believe you can do something when God promises He'll be with you . . . so here I am finding myself thinking about what information I would address to those doctors and nurses. My nurse friend, Margaret, says to tell them what my own feelings were when I was diagnosed with cancer. What were my needs? How did I want to be treated? What would I have wanted people to know then? In this conversation and in subsequent conversations with friends, I worked out an outline of what I would like to say. It would sound something like this:

VERY PERSONAL: When I thought about dying, I was very uncomfortable. I thought it could be soon. Almost nobody knew that I was alive here in Bakersfield. That fact made me feel very sad. There wouldn't be much support for my family. My kids didn't know many people. Where would my funeral be? None of the priests knew me;

who would say the Mass? How many of my family in Chicago would have the time or the financial means to come out here just to bury me. My mother was a major concern. I decided then I couldn't die . . . at the very least, I had to hold off for a while . . . now I think I'll just hold off indefinitely . . .

Karen comment: After Stanford seminar on leukemias and lymphomas—one of the best parts was that five patients spoke on their feelings. Pointed out that to them, nothing is normal. Whereas for the nurses, it's all normal. It reminded her again to be aware of the patient's point of view. Sometimes busy nurses must pride themselves on being efficient—that makes them feel pride in their accomplishment, but that doesn't do much for the patients. Dr. P's nurses reveal a lot about themselves. They present themselves as real people. Sometimes they are too much in the ordinary day-to-day things; patients have bigger crisis to deal with. One of the nicest was that Kathy told me she read my testimony (I didn't know and wasn't going to bring it up) She said she cried. That gave me a common point of discussion with her in the future; I know she knows me. I don't like to be thought of as a port, a cath, and a copy of my lab results (they all look good). Wait a minute, I feel like I'm croaking all week . . . I want to be a person attached to a family that loves me . . . so I bring photos of my family, stories of my mother, pictures of the triplets, I tell them I am writing a book . . . if they ask. Nothing much is private. I have MRI at husband's office and everybody knows I am there . . . that's one reason I put off having an enema there prior to my diagnosis. A colonoscopy was much easier for me to handle. Dr. Bhogal appointment 18 mo. later was fun. He didn't think I needed to come; he told Tony at the exam that it was granuloma; everything looked normal. I told him Ravi did not have the results. Sue Helper got them, he would correct that. He says I am doing well; you keep praying—all you have to do is pray, then you will be okay. I have another patient just like you; I saw him years later. I ran across him; he was doing fine. I was surprised. I tell you that because you want to be assured. I am telling you that so, now, you can be . . . just keep praying. I will see you in one year.

1996

HOSPICE TALK

This is the speech that she gave at the Hoffman event.
It shows the love that Mimi had for helping other people in need.

Thank you for being here tonight and sharing the unity with so many others who have lost someone they loved. Thank you for walking with that special person through his or her final journey on this earth. I know that it is both a trial and a privilege. Through tears and smiles we have all said good-bye, and tonight we remember, in a very special way the lives of a family member, a spouse, a friend, a mentor, a child . . .

We thank the dedicated people of Hoffman Hospice and unite with other hospice care workers throughout the world . . . In a sense, we are all hospice workers. We have all held a hand, shown compassion, said a prayer, and then let go. Somehow, we too become a little closer to Heaven in that moment. Part of us takes that journey with the one who has passed; part of them remains with us forever in the love beats of our hearts.

I once walked beside a mother, my friend, as she said good-bye to her 18-year-old daughter. This daughter's world had been filled with pain and suffering, yet everyday she strove to find at least one good thing. Her day began with thanks for the new dawn and the ability to move. Toward the end of her life, she gave thanks for a hand to hold as her life ebbed away. She wanted only to know that her short life had been meaningful. She did not wish for the people surrounding her to transcend the bounds of earth. She was prepared to take that final step bravely and alone. She knew the Kingdom of God awaited her. In her departure from earth, she hoped those left behind would remember her and carry on the work she was never able to complete.

I have held the hand of a friend who was dying. I have watched spousal love grow up to the moment of death. I have watched my own friends minister with care and kindness to an aging parent. I have seen the faces of the aged creased with unbearable pain, beautifully mingled with the glow of extraordinary pride in the family who surrounded them. I have seen struggle and sadness, but I witnessed great strength and an outpouring of great love. I have seen hospice workers ministering to patients at bedside, and then taking time to sit with family members and help them work through fears and concerns dealing with the natural process of dying. I have known many of the hospice staff as personal friends, and I value the compassion, caring, and quiet understanding that extends into all avenues of their lives.

I am a cancer survivor, and although I continue battling my disease and live with fear of recurrence, I have learned a new appreciation for life. In retrospect, now I would never choose to give up my cancer experience. In my difficult times, the love and care showered upon me by my family and friends was overwhelming. As my body got weaker with surgeries and chemotherapy, my heart grew larger as I felt the love and prayers of others pouring in. Though sometimes I was too weak to speak, I felt the gentle touches and I heard the loving words. I was supposed to die, and I was preparing to go willingly but sadly. I had so much to live for; God chose to let me live.

Try not to dwell too much on *why* the person you loved was taken away, but focus instead on why YOU remain. We all have a task to complete, and our love, our renewed appreciation for life, our memories, our sympathy, and our understanding can indeed make the world a better place. May God be with you and shower you with an abundance of His Blessings. May the vacant seat at your holiday table radiate the joy of a life well lived. God Bless You and Happy Thanksgiving to you all.

1996

*We get to see a glimpse into Mimi's thoughts before giv-
ing her talk at Hoffman Hospice her in a letter to her friend.*

Dear Betty,

It was great to talk to you tonight. I was figuring you'd be home
alone and just thought that would be a good time to call. It was fun—
I was just lying on our bed . . . and I got caught up on the entire St.
Louis goings on and filled you in on what's going on in my life. It is
feeling pretty good these days. I feel more like I'm in the mainstream.
I'm beginning to get involved again—different stuff but nice stuff. I'm
really starting to work pretty intensely on my book, and the Writer's
critique workshop is helping my discipline immensely.

I'm not sure if I told you this part or not—I was going to but
then my "Different Personality" came into the room to see where I'd
been hiding out for the last several hours (you know the way they do
it), and he made me forget what I was going to say. Anyway, I have
been asked to present a workshop for our Hospice here in town where I
would address the doctors and nurses. When I was first asked to do it, I
said no. Rick, the coordinator of the Celestial Correspondents program
I'm involved in, did not want to take NO for an answer. He asked why
I wouldn't do it. I said I do not like public speaking. He said, "Well,
would you lip synch for us then?" I told him I would have to consider
it seriously.

I ran the idea by Tony, whom I expected to give it a grunt (that's
what he does when he pretends he's listening but doesn't really hear),
and he said very spontaneously that he thought it could be very gratifying to me. I told Amparo I didn't know what to say. She said if I
prayed about it, the Spirit would guide me. I called my friend Margaret
who is a nurse and asked her if, as a nurse, she would want to hear a
patient's speech. She said, most definitely, she would. I asked her what
would I say, and she said tell them what you wanted and needed most
after your cancer diagnosis. I said I just wanted to be normal again,
for people to treat me normal . . . but with more UNDERSTANDING
than I had ever needed before. She said that was a perfect answer, and
I could deliver a whole workshop on it (MY NEEDS).

Then I told Margaret I would be sort of comfortable with nurses
but not talking to doctors. I couldn't do that. She laughed and said,
"Why not? You're married to one!!"

. . . and I thought, yea, that's right. They're no different than the rest of the people . . . so I'm pretty sure I'm going to do it.

In addition, my Bible Study leader says I'm articulate. I talked to my oncology nurse when I had chemo this week, and she says she just attended a seminar where five patients presented their views. She says she appreciated being reminded that EVERYTHING is new and scary for a patient. Nothing is NORMAL. She says for them, as oncology nurses who do this everyday, everything and anything is normal. So that was a valuable perspective for me. She says I should definitely do a workshop. That was sort of the final conviction. I don't know when it will be scheduled, but I'm already thinking of how to present . . . and how to pray about it . . . and how to not get nervous speaking. (One of the leaders of my Writing Critique Group wants me to go to Toast-masters with her.) I think I am going to go after I finish this course of chemo. I'm afraid if I go and get nervous while I'm on chemo, I might get diarrhea or throw-up. NOT GOOD.

I want you to know, Betty, writing this letter has fulfilled one of my writing assignments for Writer's Workshop. We must write for a half hour every single day, even if we have no inspiration. I wrote this enclosed WIG STORY (not finished yet), but I liked it . . . and now I'm waiting for my next inspiration . . .

Oh, by the way, I told you about the personality workshop I went to. I have enclosed one of the tests, and if you will take it, I will analyze it and send you a personal personality profile. I would really like to know which of the four major categories you fall into. You're a very broad-thinking person, and I see many qualities in each. The Sanguine is very outgoing and friendly. The Melancholic is very precise (which you are not in your housekeeping, but you are sooo good with recipes and sooo computer literate). The Choleric is a powerful decision maker, and I have seen you effectively take charge of many things—Playgroup, Chaminade, Travel reservations, etc. The Phlegmatic is easy going and chameleon-like, able to adapt to each of the different personalities .

If you think those names are weird, it's because they are based on Plato or Aristotle's idea that our personalities were influenced by the fluids that predominately flowed through our bodies. If you were sanguine (blood) , your heart was most powerful. If you were melancholic, your brain was most predominant. If you were choleric, the bile in your system made you irritable and you would 'put your foot down' (make decisions). If you were phlegmatic, you had a lot of mucus and were kind of laid back, looking around, and lazy (easy-going is a kinder word). What is exceptionally interesting is that once you have figured out what class you are in, you can figure out about all the people you relate to. Tony is my other personality. I am strong phlegmatic with secondary sanguine. Tony is about equally melancholic and choleric.

As I was picking through my papers looking for this test to enclose for you, I ran across the photo album you sent with our Virginia pictures in it . . . I don't know if I ever thanked you, but THANK YOU very much. It is so special . . . it'll be fun to gather our yearly collections and trace our development over the next 25 years!!! Betty, they'll be good ones . . . if we just continue to take them one day at a time. No single day can change the way we think or look or feel. We are who we are . . . and the nice thing about our present age is that we have had lots of time to develop our resilience and reflection. We have less fear and less worry because we have bounced back from lots of things we thought we couldn't handle . . . and with the grace of God we will continue to do so. With my most sincere love and prayers, I wish you a WONDERFUL BIRTHDAY!!!

P.S. Please tell Pat that I will write to her; I hope soon. I'm still working on Moses—perhaps I will send it in installments. (That Moses was a busy guy.) Pat will understand what I mean about Moses . . . has lots to do with intercessory prayer. I'm so happy to hear about John's good report.

Jan. 1998

VOLUNTEER THOUGHTS . . .

Mimi volunteered for Hoffman Hospice.
These are her thoughts for the other volunteers.

As I was putting away Christmas decorations the other day and returning to the department stores with gifts that didn't fit, I stopped for a minute to reflect on this whole season of gift giving. Gift giving makes us feel kind and thoughtful. Gift getting makes us feel special and loved. So let's carry it into the New Year . . .

I know any volunteer here at Hoffmann Hospice can show you how to do that. We specialize in giving gifts all year long. We give a few hours of our time to encourage a sick patient or relieve a devoted caregiver. We send a card or a note of encouragement or inspiration to brighten someone's day. We assist in needed office tasks. We fluff up a pillow and share a picture book. We lend an ear, a hand, or a word of understanding. We care. That's the most worthy gift of all.

In return, we receive numerous intangible gifts. We receive the satisfaction that we have helped to make someone's day a little brighter. We get a thankful sigh of relief from the busy volunteer coordinator when we say "yes." We receive a word of appreciation from an exhausted caregiver as we step in to relieve them for a couple hours. We see a smile of appreciation from a weary patient and feel a feeble hand squeeze love into our fingers. These are the best gifts for they open our hearts to more fully appreciate the wonder of life.

I like being around hearts as open as yours! Thanks for all you give.

Jan. 2002

MY LIFE

Mimi was asked to be the guest speaker at the annual Survivor's Day. This is the bio that she wrote for her introduction at that event.

Mimi Deeths is a wife and mother of four adult children. She and her husband and family moved from St. Louis, Missouri, to Bakersfield in 1991. She will confess that she found the move emotionally difficult and physically exhausting. What no one fully realized at the time was that Mimi had a progressing scoliosis in her back, a brain tumor, and the probable beginnings of colon cancer. She, however, thought life was fairly normal.

In 1992 she underwent a ten-hour back surgery, removal of seven discs, and fusions of her spine with placement of titanium rods. She spent a year in a back brace. Six months after the brace was no longer needed and life was beginning to return to normal, she was diagnosed with colon cancer already metastatic to her liver. She had a colon resection in 1994 and began chemotherapy for her colon and liver. When she spoke to her oncologist about puzzling changes in her vision, he sent her for an eye exam. MRI scans of her head revealed a brain tumor. Surgery proved that the tumor was benign. That made her think life was pretty normal again.

Four months later she had liver surgery to remove what remained of cancerous tumors in the liver. Fifteen months later a cancerous adrenal tumor was discovered and subsequently removed. She remained on chemotherapy for three more years, but a tumor grew inside her ureter, requiring cyctoscopic laser surgery in 1999. In 2001 she underwent six weeks of radiation for diffuse tumors in the area of the left adrenal bed. Currently, she is trying a combination of chemo-therapies to combat kidney and lung tumors. She's wondering how one defines normal . . .

For Mimi, normal is chemotherapy treatments, sleeping it off, and then smiling when she is able to get up. Throughout her cancer trials and tribulations, she has worked to maintain a positive attitude, setting an example of faith and grace in difficult circumstances. She has kindly and gently helped friends through their own struggles with serious illness. She has developed a strong faith in God and a deeper appreciation for His gifts. Mimi has also learned that there is probably no such thing as normal. What she does know is that God is up there watching, and she has a great team of cheerleaders down here.

June 2002

SURVIVOR'S DAY

*This is Mimi's speech from
The American Cancer Society's Annual Survivor Day.*

Thank you. Good afternoon, everyone . . . and welcome to this Survivor Day Celebration of Life.

As I listened to that introduction, I can't help but think back eight years ago. If I had known then what I was about to go through, I would never have believed that I could do it. It has not been easy, but I have had many rewards along the way. I hope that all of you here today have known those rewards—those special times of being loved and encouraged.

When I was asked a couple weeks ago to speak at Survivor's Day, I felt honored and privileged and I said, "Yes, I can do that!"

Then I went home and thought about it some more, and worried about what I would say.

I mentioned my dilemma to my friend, Richard, who is also a cancer survivor. I said, "Richard, I've been asked to speak at Survivors' Day, but I don't know what to say besides I'm poor at public speaking. I don't think I can do it."

Richard stared at me stone-faced and said, "You're right. You wouldn't be able to do that."

Somewhat deflated, I answered back, " . . . but I already told them I would.

"Well then," he said with a big grin on his face, "you will, and I think you'll be great at it!"

Richard's answer reminds me a lot about something I've learned as a cancer survivor: If we tell ourselves we can't do it, we may not be able to do it, BUT if we tell ourselves we can, there's a good chance it will happen.

You all recognize the strength of that statement—for you are survivors. You've believed, and look at what you've achieved. You've survived the diagnosis, looked over your lives, picked up the pieces, and you are in the process of moving on.

Something else I've learned is that I don't go very far without gratitude. So if you will all take a moment to bow your heads, I would like to share a short prayer with you.

Thank you, God, for bringing us together today and for all the gifts of life and healing upon the earth . . .

Thank you for all the committee members, medical staffs, and families and friends who support us by loving us and working so hard to help us remember and retain this precious gift of life . . .

Now I ask God to bless the words that flow from my mouth so that they will glorify Him and bring encouragement and blessings to all the people assembled here, my fellow cancer survivors and all our families and friends. Amen.

Now back to that speech I told Richard I was going to do. As I began to prepare it last week, I got excited about it. My mind went off in a hundred different directions. I remembered a story I wanted to tell you, but I couldn't get it to tie in with my message . . . then I got to where I wasn't sure what my message was. Then on Wednesday, I had chemotherapy all day, flaked out for a couple days after that, and got completely behind in my task. What do you say at Survivors' Day anyway?

So yesterday, in total frustration, I said to my family gathered in the den, "Okay. I have a problem. In twenty four hours I need to deliver a talk. I don't know what I'm going to say or how I'm going to say it. What should I do?"

My husband Tony is a man of few words, but when he does speak, he shows great insight. I like to call it wisdom. Well, he sat back in his chair and said, "Why don't you put a phone in your hand and pretend you are talking to someone newly diagnosed with cancer. You're good at that."

I took that as the compliment it was meant to be. One of the things I have learned about being a survivor is to graciously accept compliments and affirmations. When we are struggling, it's so important to learn to love yourself.

In the beginning of my cancer diagnosis, I found it hard to love myself. I felt guilty that I was ruining the lives of my family members, destroying their sense of security. I was afraid and felt like a coward. I felt like friends would drift away for I had nothing to contribute anymore. I felt like a huge obstacle had just been placed in my life plan.

That reminds me of a story I want to share with you because it taught me a powerful lesson. This is how the story goes . . .

God made a man and allowed the man to choose from among a variety of tasks the one that he was willing perform. Upon looking at the objects connected to each task, the man chose the boulder. It was a very large rock as tall as the man and just as hefty in its width.

The man's task, God then explained to him, was simply to push the rock.

So the next morning the man got up at sunrise and he began pushing. He pushed with all his might, all day long in the hot sun. The rock did not move. By nightfall he was exhausted and he went to bed.

Faithful, to the task the man got up the next morning and pushed some more. He used his arms. He used his thighs. He wedged his leg between it and gave his leg a powerful kick thrust. The rock remained. He did this all day until he became exhausted. Night fell. He went to bed.

But the next morning the man got up. Today he would butt-up against the rock with his shoulders and lean into it with all his might. Even that grew tiresome, but the man persevered. The rock, however, still didn't move. By nightfall, he dropped like that boulder into his bed.

Once again, he awoke early the next morning. Today he braced his back against the rock and pushed with all the power in his flat back with the strength of his thighs and his legs. Still again the rock did not move.

Finally, in desperation, the man cried out to God, " God, I cannot get this rock to move. I have tried my arms. I have tried my thighs and legs. I have tried my shoulders until the skin has worn thin. I have tried my back. I can't move it! "

God listened to the man and answered him, "Who said anything about MOVING the rock. I only asked you to PUSH it. Now stand back here for a minute. Let me look at you. You have done the task I have asked. Look what you have accomplished by obedience. Your arms have grown well muscled. Your chest and lungs are more powerful. Your legs and thighs are much stronger than they were before. Look at the development in your shoulders and chest. The condition of your heart is better than ever. You have met my challenge with the right attitude. Well done, my son."

Like the man in the story, I want to do things beyond what I am asked to do. When I was diagnosed with cancer eight years ago, the task I wanted to accomplish was reaching remission. For several years,

I became discouraged when that didn't happen. I thought I had failed at my task, and I called out to God in my frustration. His answer was clear. He showed me the strengths I had developed. I am doing just what He wants with my life. I have grown. I have developed. I have become stronger. I am doing the best that I can do.

I have learned that I am not alone in this journey through life. God has given me His Word. I have the love of my family, the support of my friends, the wisdom of the medical profession, and people like you to inspire and encourage me with your survivor stories.

I have grown more confident as the woman I now am and not in the woman I dreamed I would be.

I have learned that asking "Why?" brings no answer, but asking "How?" can bring a compassionate response.

I saw my worth when I understood that my experience could provide a source of strength and hope for others survivors.

I have learned that success is in the doing, not in the getting; in the trying, not in the triumph.

I learned that Joy is available to everyone, but you can't necessarily expect it to come and find you. Sometimes, you have to go look for it. Sometimes, it happens when you are pushing your hardest on the big boulders of life.

So remember, when you are facing your biggest challenges and being tested and toned, it's not necessarily the moving that matters, but Just Keep On Pushing.

Congratulations on being strivers; that's what makes you Survivors.

May God bless you with success.

CHAPTER 9

Relay For Life

Faithful, loyal, kind, compassionate, considerate, loving, happy, thoughtful, caring, helpful, trustworthy, reliable, devoted, joyful, cheerful, unselfish, admired, prayerful, loved God, her family & friends. These are just a few words that begin to describe the type of person that Mimi was made of. Mimi never met a stranger! I was introduced to Mimi through Dr. Ravi Patel, and from there, a wonderful bond developed. The gentle and kind spirit that Mimi possessed was so incredible to me, and I admired her tremendously. It never ceased to amaze me that when she was at CBCC, no matter how she was feeling, she was never without a smile, hugs, and encouraging words for others.

As our friendship grew, there was something very special about Mimi, and I felt the Lord placed it upon my heart to pray for her on a daily basis. This is something I wanted my children to be a part of as well. Before they went to bed every night, they prayed for Mimi even though they had not met her yet. It was a Relay for Life event that brought my children and Mimi together for the first time. We were setting up our CBCC campsite at the Relay, and Mimi had come by to see how everyone was doing. It was at that time that I asked my oldest daughter, Madison, who we prayed for each night. She replied, "Mimi Deeths," and it was then that I introduced her to Mimi and a special relationship was formed. From that point on, the Relay for Life had a different and special meaning and was never the same again!

It is so hard to put into words the wonderful feelings and emotions that we shared with Mimi. Some of the best memories are the times we shared at the park, watching the girls play as Mimi and I visited and reminisced about our families. Some of the most special times were at the Relay for Life and are memories I will hold onto for a lifetime ~ my favorite being Madison snuggled up in Mimi's lap, sound asleep during an evening event. She always brought a smile to my girls' faces with the special and thoughtful gifts she would give them. She would even surprise them in her thoughtful ways with special gifts in the mail when they least expected it, and they always included special notes to each of them. The only way to fully describe Mimi is to say that she was truly and definitely a "one-of-a-kind" individual and someone I strive to emulate.

There is not a day that goes by that Mimi is not brought up by either Madison or McKenzie, and she is still prayed for every night by my girls in their prayers. The times we spent with Mimi, in addition to all of our fond memories, are without a doubt very cherished. Unaware of what I was asked to do, one night I asked my oldest daughter, Madison (7), to tell me in her own words what Mimi meant to her. Her exact words were, "She meant everything to me. She was very loving & sweet, kind, faithful, and fun. She was a blessing to me and had the most awesome and loving heart that Jesus created!"

We love and miss you Mimi. Your presence will always be in our hearts!

Debbie Davis
Friend and secretary at CBCC

May 2001

HEALING HANDS AND HAPPY HEARTS

This is a story about Mimi's special little friend Madison. Every time Madison saw Mimi, her face lit up. Two weeks before Mimi died, Debbie brought Madison over to read a story to Mimi. Madison was so excited that she could hardly contain herself. It was a very special time for them both.

Madison, being 4 years old, knew her prayer pattern well. She prayed them in her specific order every night as she sat beside her mother just before going to sleep. Months ago, mom had taught her to add a few special petitions for the health of certain patients she had encountered in her job at a cancer center.

So little Madison faithfully prayed each night, "Please God to put your healing hands on Mimi Deeths, Ella Pedroza, and Marilyn Pruitt." Madison didn't know these patients personally, or if she had met them, she had forgotten who they were as the playful days of childhood colored the brief memory of any on-the-spot adult introductions.

One night after weeks of praying for this trio of cancer survivors, the child's mother, Debbie, curiously asked, "Madison, do you remember who these people are?"

'Yes, I know!" she said with sparkling certainty. "They're my dolls' names!"

Madison continued to play with her dolls everyday and imagined them very alive and having such wonderful fun. Every night, she prayed and imagined God laying His big healing hands on Mimi Deeths, Ella Pedroza, and Marilyn Pruitt.

Fantasy and reality mix so smoothly in the crystal simplicity of a 4-year-old's mind that only Madison knew of the magical relationship between the daytime dolls with whom she played and the nighttime names for whom she prayed. Occasionally, an adult will be gifted to share in a child's magic for mixing wishes and reality when they walk into the child's world.

I was enchanted when I walked into Madison's world at the American Cancer Society's Ninth Annual Relay for Life in Bakersfield, California. She was there "helping" her mom and Nana set up the Cancer Center's campsite. I had heard from her mother and grandmother that little Madison remembered me and a couple other patients in her prayers every night, and my heart was warmed hearing about this thoughtful little girl. When I met her that evening, Madison was holding on to her mother's hand, as Debbie and I greeted one another. Then Debbie bent down to her daughter's eye level, and I stooped down to look more closely at this charming child as her mother asked, "Madison, do you know who this is?"

Madison looked puzzled and then answered, "No, who is she?"

"This is Mimi Deeths," said her mom.

Little Madison's eyes glimmered, her mouth opened in wide surprise, and her mind went into wonderland, as her little arms flew around my neck and she quietly and curiously exclaimed, "Yooou're Mee Mee Deeths?!" Tears were forming in my eyes, as I felt her excited little heart pounding against mine. "Are your two other friends with you?" she asked excitedly.

I began to question who she meant, and then quickly calculated the logical assumption that since their names were prayed right along with mine that I must know the other two women from her nightly prayers. I told her we were all friends of her Mommy, but I didn't know the other ladies. She wondered out loud if they would come later. I said that maybe they would come, and I sensed the eager anticipation of that possibility in her eyes. Then she stared into my eyes and ever so gently began stroking my face, "But, how did you get healed from your disease?"

I could only answer, "Because God wants me to feel better now, and you help Him to remember every night with your prayers. Those prayers are very special to me and to God. Thank you for saying them."

With one more big hug, Madison kissed me and then ran off to play Follow the Leader with June-Bug. I was the one left in wide-eyed wonder with a look of enchantment on my face.

———

Jesus said, " Let the little children come to Me, and do not hinder them, for the kingdom of God belongs to such as these. I tell you the truth, anyone who will not receive the Kingdom of God like a little child will never enter it." And He took the little children in his arms, put his hands on them and blessed them.
Mark 10:14–16

2002

THE GIFT

The Relay For Life is the American Cancer Society's big annual fundraiser. It is a 24-hour event in which teams participate and walk around a track for 24 hours. One member of the team must be on the track at all times. The Bakersfield event is one of the largest in the nation. In 2003, over $1 million was raised.

Saturday morning, April 27, 2002, is crisp and cool. Excitement is in the air. Banners, balloons, decorated campsites, a large sound stage, and thousands of people are gathering around the front of the stage on the California State Bakersfield campus for the first lap of the American Cancer Society's Relay for Life. I am proudly wearing my survivors T-shirt, which is given out free of charge to all survivors. The shirts have our American flag on the front with a star and the word "Survivor" printed down the front side. Seeing these shirts on so many people reminds me just how much community support lies behind this event. The shirts separate the team of survivors from the loving compassionate friends and family now beginning to line the field.

This is the third time I have participated in the Relay, and this scene, which I have often tried to describe to others, is being shared for the first time with several new survivors whom I have met recently. Most especially, however, this is the first time my daughter, Liz, who recently graduated from college, has been in town and able to come and watch. I'm really excited now for her to see this event I have tried to describe to her. Liz's being here reminds me again of her high school years with the excitement and the roar of the crowd as I sat in the bleachers during her volleyball and basketball games. I always loved the cheers and high hopes for the home team, flooding the hearts of all the spectators. Today is different—I am on that home team with at least 800 other cancer survivors in their T-shirts. Impromptu photos taken with my little camera will try to capture the unique joy and sharing of this day, but photos will be inadequate. The emotions and feelings lie too deeply imprinted upon the heart to be fairly reflected, even in the smiling eyes.

At 9:00 A.M. the loudspeaker calls for the line up of the cancer survivors on the track. Liz recedes into the background of the grassy field with our friends, John and Marcia, who have awakened especially for their first experience of witnessing this event. They stand together and watch the activity happening on the track. T-shirted survivors line up ten and twelve abreast across the width of the track. Approximately 800 strong, we extended 80 layers deep down the length of the track. Those numbers speak of hope. In this current day of technology and improved medicines for oncology, we are alive! Bald heads, wigs, wheelchairs, scars, smiles and strength—we each have our story.

No story, however, stands out as brave, bold, and optimistic as the line leaders' story. Leading the army of survivors is the bright red, antique fire engine, holding a most precious cargo—the cancer kids! These sturdy little survivors, with their range of shy to smiling faces, prove that the love lavished on them is stronger than the disease that threatens to destroy them. Especially appropriate to the Relay this year is the patriotic theme. We celebrate and mourn, too, the brave firemen in the wake of our country's September 11 suffering. Today we have our firemen driving their fire truck, helping our children have courage and feel proud. I see heroes honoring heroes. Everyone is moved by this sight.

Then thousands of voices strong, the entire field joins in singing "America the Beautiful" with our favorite local television news team of Robin Mangarin and Jim Scott. We really feel the words. We dream of a day when those little children, high up in the fire truck, will know America, will walk as adults, where we are now, in a world without cancer. We feel it happening . . .

I hear this familiar line beautifully sung over the loudspeaker . . ."America, America, God shed His grace on thee . . ." My mind drifts heavenward and automatically substitutes "God shed His grace on *me*" because I have known His miracles so often. I'm into a personal prayer of thanksgiving here. A tear rolls down my face.

The song continues, "And crowned thy good with brotherhood from sea to shining sea . . ." Now I am back to the moment. I'm part of the crowd. We are a "brotherhood" of cancer survivors who see a community of supporters surrounding us, lining the length of the field it seems "from sea to shining sea." I look for the faces of my daughter and my friends in the crowd. It's too packed to see them, and we are now directed to bow our heads in prayer.

I am alone with my God now as the invocation, sensitively spoken for all to hear over the sound system, provokes an overwhelming feeling of gratitude for life and a deep feeling of loss for those whose hands we have held here in years gone by. We feel appreciation, faith, love, unity, hope, and a mixture of emotions that causes our Spirit to soar. The prayer is ended, hands are joined and raised in victory and praise, and soon we are walking down the track . . . almost in a trance . . . as cheers and shouts and smiles of encouragement surround us.

Today I have forgotten that some days are a struggle as I go through chemotherapy and its side effects. I'm walking within a crowd of optimistic people who fill me with strength. I'm not an individual. I'm part of a team. In my marching mode, suddenly I hear the voice of my friend break through my thoughts and she says, "Mimi, your daughter needs you." I look to the right and directly in front of me. Five or six fellow survivors walk beside me separating me from the face of love that I see. I am frozen in the moment. The crowd marches on, but I stand still.

I see the face of my daughter, Liz, breaking away from the line of standing spectators. Unharnessed tears flood down her cheeks. Initially hesitant, she, now with determined strides, makes her way to where I wait. I am frozen, misty eyed, in the center of the track. I feel the past eight years of pain for cancer's uncertainty, which I never wanted my children to know, but then I see the love, the undying hope, and the pride in my daughter's face. Emotions spill over in rivulets of tears as we smother, embraced in each other's arms and openly weep as our hearts beat together. In this moment, I am holding a life so precious I cannot describe it. I hold my baby, the little girl who loves me, the teenager who feared I could die, who held my hand through numerous recovery times, and now is an adult devoting her professional life to healthcare. This is one of life's magic moments. In this moment, I understand that she carries my whole family's shared feelings for me— the love, the pain, the concern, the compassion, the fears of loss, the courage to move through this. It's what I've come to know as a sacred moment, when you know that God has blessed it from the beginning. I have never walked alone. I never will. I know beyond any shadow of doubt that I will continue to hold on to the hand of God, the love of my family, the care of my physicians and staff, and the support of my friends. This is a day of renewed conviction.

Liz and I walk the track, hand in hand together for a few paces, savoring the moment. Our love turns into a bit of laughter, as Liz lets loose of my hand and then says sheepishly, "I think I better go back to my place now," and she slips back to her spectator spot. On the track, life marches on as the ranks of survivors continue to pass. I hasten my pace to catch up with the friends who have moved on ahead. I need to reach them to pass this energy on. My heart is bursting, for I know God has chosen the circumstances, the messenger, and the moment to display His intimacy with me, to breathe life into the message that "Faith, hope, and love remain, but the greatest of these is love (1 Corinthians 13:13)."

1999

RELAY FOR LIFE I

*Mimi participated in and raised money for the
Relay For Life for several years.
This is her letter from 1999.*

Tony and I and our family were relative newcomers to Bakersfield when I was diagnosed almost five years ago with metastatic colon cancer. When I look back, I never cease to be amazed by the support and concern shown to us by the Bakersfield community. The medical community was outstanding in their efficient networking system of quality care covering my myriad problems. Neighbors and friends were most generous and compassionate in helping us get back on track with our lives. God held my hand (Isaiah 41:13).

Now I feel I have an opportunity to give some of that back to the community. On Saturday, April 24, I will be participating in the American Cancer Society's RELAY FOR LIFE. I've never done it before, so I can't really tell you a whole lot about it. My friends who have been involved, however, say it is a very heartwarming and fun day.

The way the relay works is like this: Local organizations and corporations organize a relay team consisting of 10–24 members. I understand that last year there were about 40 teams. The relay is a 24-hour affair so there are team campsites set up around the track. At least one person from each team MUST be on the track at all times during the 24-hour period. (I'm not taking a night shift!)

When I heard that you didn't have to run or be fast, I figured this was something I could do. I'll be joining a team from the **Comprehensive Blood and Cancer Center** since I've come to know and appreciate the people over there on my weekly sojourns . . .

Now **if you are not on a relay**, I have an **opportunity** for you to participate. You don't need to run or walk. In fact, you don't even have to be there! If you make a donation to the American Society, I will carry your name in my pocket as I walk around the track . . . and you can just feel good about that.

I'm sending a lot of these letters to unsuspecting friends, so no one needs to feel obliged to send in a large donation—$5.00, $10.00, $20.00 from many people adds up to a sizeable amount that will help greatly in cancer research and patient care. I need my personal **dona-**

tions in by April 5 so I have enclosed a self-addressed envelope and return card for your convenience. Please request a receipt if you wish. I'll send a report of my experience with the relay and a personal thank you soon after the event. (Tony says if you send an extra five dollars, I promise not to send you a copy of my report.)

I thank you in advance for your consideration. This event, which will be held in the Garces Memorial Stadium from 9 A.M. on Saturday, April 24 until 9 A.M. on Sunday, April 25, is open to the public. There will be food booths, fancy tents, and fun people. We'd love to have you cheer us on . . . so come on over if you can.

RELAY FOR LIFE II

This is another letter for the Relay from the same year. No one knows why there are two drafts, but they are both good.

Dear

I have a plan . . . and I would really appreciate your helping me carry it out.

You see, I sit having intravenous chemotherapy each week for a couple hours. I've been doing it for almost five years now, so I'm used to it and find that it provides me with some valuable thinking time. I don't much like the side effects of the treatment, but I do appreciate the benefits it has provided for me—it has given me a second chance at life! That's a gift I shall never take for granted.

I have been so blessed with Faith . . . and family, friends, and physicians, like you, who encourage me by their presence and their prayers. I am fortunate to have medical insurance that covers most of my medical care but have become increasingly aware of the hardship a disease like cancer causes for so many families.

I have seized an opportunity to help them, and I am excited that this year I am able to participate in the American Cancer Society's RELAY FOR LIFE. The RELAY is held each year here in Bakersfield at the Garces Memorial Track. This year the 24-hour event will be from Saturday at 9:00 A.M. until Sunday 9 A.M. on April 24 and 25. Approximately forty teams are expected to set up their campsites and get involved in this community service. Each team consists of a minimum of 10 people, with each member collecting at least $100.00 in donations—that being accomplished, the 24-hour marathon begins . . . Each team is required to have at least one person run (walk, waddle, crawl, roll in a wheel chair, whatever) on the track at all times. Speed is not the object of the race—team spirit is all it takes.

I will be on a very spirited team from the Comprehensive Blood and Cancer Center. My oncology buddies—doctors, nurses, staff, and cancer survivors—are planning for a great time with friendly camaraderie and a carnival atmosphere surrounding this sincere service project. The first lap of the day will consist only of cancer survivors. A Saturday evening ceremony will light our little corner of Bakersfield with luminaries, each one dedicated to the honor or memory of a loved one affected by cancer.

I ask you, my friends, for a small contribution. I'm sending out 100 requests—so your five, ten, or twenty dollar donations will add up to great strides in cancer research and patient support. I must have all my contributions in by April 5, so if you are able to help, please return the little envelope and card enclosed as soon as possible. If you can't send money now, please return the card anyway with your good wishes and prayers. That would be a wonderful gift.

I will carry my collection of cards as I walk along . . . and I will be grateful for your thoughtfulness, and thank God that you are my friend. May God bless you.

1999

AWE

Mimi had an outpouring of responses.

I was going to wait until the Relay for Life was over, and then send out thank-you notes and a review of my experiences as a first-time participant. However, your responses to my request have been so overwhelming that I have to write a thank-you now . . .

My goal was to send out 100 letters. I reached my goal with 60 of them going to family and friends out of town and 40 going to physicians and friends right here in Bakersfield. I sent out 100 empty, self-addressed return envelopes . . . and I cried as I began to open the ones returned to me. They were filled with generous contributions given from the bottom of your hearts, I know . . . and they were filled with so much love, concern, and encouragement that I cannot even begin to express my gratitude and deep appreciation for your thoughtfulness.

I had hoped for ten and twenty dollar checks so I could feel supported in my endeavor to assist the American Cancer Society. I got so much more. Thank you for your generosity and your loving expressions of encouragement. May God Bless you as you have blessed me.

I hope you had a beautiful Easter celebration . . . and please take time this spring to smell the flowers.

RACE FOR THE CURE

This was the letter Mimi sent out after the event.

May 27,1999

Dear

Well, I promised you that I would send you a RELAY FOR LIFE update soon after the event was over. I hope you think a month later qualifies as "soon."

I'll start by saying it was A RAINBOW DAY that I will never forget.

I hardly slept the night before . . . because I was excited about the team shirt I had received the day before. Our team consisted of eighty doctors, nurses, staff, and patients from the Comprehensive Blood and Cancer Center. We were all going to be wearing hunter green golf shirts with a checkered flag logo on the front designating us as Pit Crew. The back of the shirt had a big bright yellow race car decaled with the cancer center logo and #1. Our theme arranged in a rainbow above the car proclaimed "Racing For The Cure." Our campsite for the weekend was fixed up like a racing car, pit change area, which is where we hung out to relax between the events going on all day and night on the grandstand stage.

Eighty-three other teams were displaying their themes in multi-colored shirts—like the battleship campsite from the Wheeler Radiation Oncology Center with their sailor shirts and hats, mops and buckets—and the theme "Mop out Cancer." A team of ten high school girls covered their tent in bamboo, Hawaiian style, and made a big, paper-mache volcano in front of it with the theme *Kileau Cancer* (play on words—Kill ya' cancer). There was another campsite with a soccer goal net set up where participants could try for a goal. The theme: "Kick Cancer." It was fun just to walk around the campsites and look at them.

I had all my notes of encouragement from family and friends (my love notes) in the pocket of my jeans as the first lap of the race began at 9:00 A.M. on Saturday morning, April 24. The public address system called for all cancer survivors to line up at the starting line. We were all given blue T-shirts that read 1999 Relay For Life. The back had the words "Proud Cancer Survivor" spelled out on it. Leading the first lap was a big, red fire engine with all the children surviving cancer waving as they went. It was the Rose Parade in miniature—wonderful! It was inspiring to see those little kids, and I was preoccupied watching them as I walked along behind the fire engine. Then I realized that a crowd about 2,000 strong had all left their tent dwellings and stood lining the track clapping and cheering for us as we floated through the Survivor's Lap. It was a jubilant time.

Twelve hours later, in the dark at 9 P.M., we would walk that same track after an exciting but exhausting day. Only this time, cancer survivors were joined by the entire community as we slowly processed around the track and read the names on the 5,000-plus luminaries listing cancer survivors and loved ones who have succumbed to the disease. This was a very reflective and reverent time. I had lit many luminaries for friends and family members . . . and I felt like they were all there with me in the dark of night. Sometimes, I felt sad but never alone. Many people had lit luminaries with my name on them. They made me smile and my heart beat faster to send out all the love I felt. By the end of the night I was exhausted . . . and overwhelmed.

I am not used to twelve-hour days with lots of activity. Chemotherapy makes me feel like an old lady much of the time—but this day was different. I had all my friends and family members in my pocket and on the field with me. I do like to party . . . and I did. I did my assigned laps of the relay—probably walked about five miles that day. Massage therapists had volunteered to give massages all day long, and they had their massage tables set up in their tent. (The theme: Rub Out Cancer, of course.) We went over there to take a nap!

There was a country line dance instructor on stage, giving line-dance lessons. With two hundred people lined up on the grass for lessons, I figured I could sneak my uncoordinated self in for some lessons, so I went with a couple friends and we line danced for 45 minutes. It was great fun . . . and nobody noticed (or cared) if you missed some steps. After that, there was a 30-minute kickboxing demonstration. I chose to be in the audience for that one and just laugh—I'd never seen that routine before. Following that there was some swing dancing—again, I chose to watch, but what fun!!!

All this took place under a beautiful, blue sky; the weather could not have been more perfect! There were skits, inspirational speakers, awards, live bands, a disc jockey, and a track with thousands of rainbow shirted people walking for a great cause. Free food was provided all day (and night) by local sponsors. I didn't stay the night—I knew I would have been a party pooper . . . and the thought of a night's sleep on the hard ground did not seem conducive to being able to get up and actually walk the next day!

Anyway, I needed to go home for the night and nestle with Tony. The day had been overwhelming. You know how I sent you those letters after the donations came in??? Well, I was shocked at the amount of donations I collected . . . and so was the Relay for Life committee. I collected over $4,000 from my family and friends (Christmas card list). Local physicians and friends from the cancer center added several thousand more. Our team was called to the stage and awarded first place TEAM in contributions collected. I was asked to remain on stage after that. When my oncologist took the microphone and started speaking about a person who was fighting the cancer battle courageously, going out of her way to help others by collecting funds, and had recently become a published author, I knew he was going to say my name . . .

I wanted to point out to him that so many other people here are courageous and that all I did was ask for donations and **other people** gave them to me and that all I had was two pages in a recently published book (*Encouraging Hands, Encouraging Hearts* by Linda Evans Shepherd, pages 150–152) . . . except right then, the whole field started to clap . . . and I was awarded a big, blue ribbon for being the individual collecting the largest amount of contributions, given a RELAY FOR LIFE logo blanket, and gift certificates. Then I was handed the microphone . . . I had your love notes in my pocket; my friends were smiling up at me from the field. I don't remember all I said, but I know it ended with the words, "With the kind of love and support that I have, it's possible to do anything . . ." The people clapped. I heard you clapping too. Thank you and may God bless you as I have been blessed.

April 2001

FOUNTAIN OF LIFE

Linda is one of Dr. Patel's secretaries who Mimi became close friends with over the years. This was written after a Relay For Life.

April 30, 2001

Dear Linda,

Congratulations and thank you for all the thought, time, effort, and emotion you put into developing and setting up the campsite for this year's Relay for Life. I thought it was most appropriate that you brought the symbolism of the Fountain of Life to our campsite. During this past year, the fountain has been a meaningful and beautiful addition to the entry of the Cancer Center, and I think it was very appropriate to tie in the Center itself with our campsite theme.

For our dedicated staff, patients, and their families, our Comprehensive Blood and Cancer Center represents all the themes displayed on the Wall of Reflection, which was caringly constructed for our site. The fresh flowers added color and the warm feeling of eternal spring. Indeed, it provided a quiet place where people came respectfully to reflect or to gain more information about controlling and treating cancer. The words, FAITH, LOVE, HOPE, LIFE, HEALING, and COURAGE are truly the finest and most complete summary of the primary inspiration in the minds and hearts of those struggling with cancer and their caregivers. The photos of survivors and staff were a powerful reminder of how real cancer is. The site and theme very sensitively epitomized what the RELAY FOR LIFE stands for—compassionate treatment, continual research, and the hope that someday there will be no more photos needed on that wall.

I am proud of how our excellent Cancer Center has enhanced services available to our community, and I am very grateful for the encouragement, energy, and devotion of the entire staff. I truly feel that I was able to participate in the RELAY FOR LIFE again this year because of the efforts of the doctors and support staff dedicated to keeping me alive. I know many, many others share this sincere view for themselves and their loved ones.

Were we disappointed that our campsite did not obtain even an honorable mention? We shouldn't be. The point was not the prize of recognition. The judging committee had certain criteria that they sought based on mere human intellect and opinion. Our campsite was based on the cooperatively woven hearts and emotions of both patients and staff. Those qualities surpass technical judgment. The wall and the fountain of life meant what they needed to mean to each person who walked through.

Because of the sensitive impact of our display and the very serious reality of cancer in our day, I think that the photo wall with the fountain of life in the foreground should become a permanent theme at the RELAY FOR LIFE. A great deal of time and careful construction went into the development of our site. The walls will continue to stand for future years. Let the photos be updated for next year, but I don't see how you could ever improve on the theme.

Thank you and your dedicated committee for your lovely and heartwarming idea of what the RELAY FOR LIFE should continue to portray. Our campsite will always be Number One in my heart and soul.

I will proudly wear my shirt and proclaim its message. Thank you once again for all your effort.

Sincerely,

CHAPTER 10

Compassion

My friend, Mimi, was one of the most giving people I have ever known. I will always treasure her mentoring and sense of humor.

When it became obvious that Mimi would soon be going home to our Father, I would be delighted when her family would ask me to sit with her. At last I thought I could do something for her. We shared many tender moments—laughing , crying, and talking about dying. Finally, I was able to give to her, but in Mimi's true style, she ended up giving me her greatest gift. I was called to work with the dying and their families through hospice care—even after death she is still present to us.

Mary Richard
Friend

1996

KATIE'S WINGS

Mimi wrote this after dropping Katie off at medical school.
It expresses Mimi's love for her daughter Katie and
Katie's love and concern for her mother.

In early August Tony and I left Katie and David standing together and waving us off as we exited Parking lot #30 at Irvine. We were tired and hot after a day of helping Katie move into her new, campus apartment. I was trying to be tough, as Tony looked back at the kids and said, "I feel like I'm abandoning my children." I looked back at our two adult children, smiling and waving enthusiastically by the U-Haul van and thought what a "softie" their Dad was. Those kids didn't look abandoned to me—they were ready to move on with the excitement of their youthful lives. I was so proud of the two of them. I thought my heart would burst . . .

Then my tears came just before we turned to hit Adobe Circle Drive. Katie wouldn't be with me tomorrow when we procrastinated over a cup of morning coffee. Her stroke across my shoulder as I lay sick in bed would no longer wake me gently in the aftermath of chemotherapy as she came in and questioned, "How 'ya doin,' Little Buddy?" Her friendly personality, her honesty, her funny way of saying serious things, and her sensitivity would be sorely missed in our home. She had come home for a year to help me heal, and near as I could tell, her mission had been accomplished.

I was now six weeks postop from adrenal gland surgery for a second metastatic tumor, and my prognosis was looking pretty positive. Now it was her turn to bloom, to use what she had learned, and to steer her own course toward the rest of her life. She never failed to give. I only know, truly, how she gave to me. From the responses I see in the rest of her family and her myriad friends, I know she gives similarly to everyone.

Katie found a way to make it back and forth from San Diego to L.A. in a one-day, round trip on the day of my back surgery, to spend much of the ten hours with her dad as they waited for me to emerge from anesthesia, to be there when I woke up at 10 P.M., and then to head back to school for classes the next morning. Months later, she was able to confront my diagnosis of metastatic colon cancer over the phone, compose herself sufficiently to end her school year in San Diego, and then come home to truly celebrate my birthday in the hospital, and help to give me the conviction to battle my infirmity. Katie seemed to understand a sick person's need to be "normal" as she brought Bree home for Thanksgiving, and they took their rotation, Pepsi's in hand, in party mode, around my hospital bed following brain surgery in 1994. She was the one who freed up her time to oversee my move from ICU to a room at UCLA following liver surgery, when Tony was called back to Bakersfield to work. Then this summer, she was there again along with the rest of the family, back at UCLA in June as I awoke from the adrenal surgery. She had taken time off from work to stay with me. Again, I celebrated another birthday in the hospital, but her small gift to me, the little, wooden, happy massager with the smiley face tied up in ribbons and delivered in the form of a hospital bed, back massage, came with such love and tenderness that the feeling it gave me is impossible to describe. I'll miss her warm fuzziness at home . . .

. . . And that is why it is hard to send my daughter off to medical school, but it is also why it is easy to let her go. She has so much to offer the world. Her conviction is based upon much personal experience, modeling of her father and sister who chose medicine, and the soul searching that her seeking spirit demands. I'm proud to say that her roots are well established. I feel them in my heart. Now she needs the wings to fly. God will be her guide. I feel that deeply in my soul.

1997

ACT OF KINDNESS

*This story shows how the simple kindness of one person
can impact multiple people.*

"If one part (of the body of Christ) suffers,
all parts suffer with it; if one
part is honored,
every part rejoices with it."
1 Corinthians 12:26

As a wife and mother with a hard-working, busy husband and four young adult children, I sometimes find it hard to handle my long-term illness. In June of 1994, I was diagnosed with metastatic colon cancer and sometimes am disappointed that I can't keep up with my family members the way I used to do. Whereas I used to organize and plan, now with chemotherapy and its side effects, I have to sort of wing it day-to-day. Sometimes, I get discouraged that I can't be the wife and mother whom I used to be. I have always enjoyed my role as caretaker and comforter, and now it seems too often I am the one being cared for and comforted. I am bothered sometimes that my husband and children must enter into their normal work and college stresses compounded by the additional concern for me.

When I get frustrated by my condition, however, I recall the many kindnesses to me that have been freely given. I remind myself of the watchful eye of God who healed me after so many surgeries, the compassion of the doctors who have cared for me, the patience and maturity of my family as they have learned to cope, the visits, cards, and prayers so lovingly offered by friends. Through each of them, I understand the integration of all the members of the Mystical Body of Christ, and this comprehension is awesome. The ways the stronger members have supported me in my weakness are so numerous that I can not even count them, but one incident particularly stands out in my mind.

In January of 1995, I was hospitalized for complications from the side effects of a chemotherapy, fever, dehydration, and mental confusion. I was concerned for my 17-year-old daughter, Elizabeth, who was scheduled to leave town that week for a school varsity basketball tournament. She had been excited about this for weeks and had arranged to do the required academic assignments for the school days she would be missing. Now, however, because of my precarious medical condition, she was torn between staying in town and going to her basketball tournament.

On the early morning of their departure, Liz was dropped off with all her gear at the school parking lot. As the other team members arrived, they kissed their parents good-bye and excitedly gathered into the school district van. Then the coach climbed into the driver's seat and headed out of town with the van full of sleepy, high school girls. He took one detour before heading to the highway. At 8:00 A.M. he pulled into the hospital parking lot, stopped at the front door, and called to Liz to jump out, go in, and kiss her mother good-bye.

Liz bounded out, rushed up to my room, and gave me a big bear hug and kiss good-bye. That is the best medicine any mother could hope for! My spirits soared as she excitedly exited my room to reboard the van. Just thinking about that early morning encounter made me smile for the rest of the day.

It is truly amazing what a tiny action from a caring person can do. Though my daughter delivered the kiss, it was the coach who took the detour, which delighted our day. His stopping by that morning relieved my daughter's silent, unspoken fears. Being acknowledged in such a thoughtful way by her coach increased her already strong admiration for him. In addition, the coach had taught all the girls an important strategy off the basketball court. He had shown them the art of compassion. He had opened the door so these young women could be responsive to a friend in need. They showed their concern for Liz when she reentered the van and understood the emotional turmoil she was suffering in silence. They could live the Mystical Body of Christ, where the healthy members care for the hurting one. They became teammates in the game of life. In addition, this interaction reminded the girls to honor their own parents, just as God's people were ordered to do in the Ten Commandments.

My daughter and I are both lucky to be on the receiving end of this lovely act of kindness. It has made us both better people as we try to remember to take that fifteen-minute detour to care for each other and to teach the lessons of Jesus Christ.

Mid-2001

MY FLOWER FRIEND

This poem was written as a thank-you note to Mimi's friends.

She came with a poinsettia just before Christmas,
ducked into our den where I was taking a rest,
Left a kiss on my cheek and a smile in my heart,
Then as quickly as she came, she had to depart. . . . .

She had other homes in which to share her cheer
Ignoring the amorphous burden she had to bear,
Her mission was to bring beauty and see others smile,
Again she would stay just a little while.

And the plant she left behind would brighten our holidays
And recall to us Judith's "Norwegian elf" ways.
With leaves of red, pink, white, and green—
This was truly the most beautiful poinsettia we'd ever seen!

When that weekend was ended, and Monday arrived,
There came bad news for which we cried.
Breast cancer had been discovered in our loving elf—
We would help her feel strong when she wondered about herself!

Matt encouraged her, and the kids homeward drove,
And Judith began chemotherapy, surrounded by love.
By Christmas she was sick, but not forlorn,
As she was surrounded by family and friends, and Jesus was born.

At times like this our convictions are made strong,
As we hold onto the hands of others and walk along.
And keep our eyes turned heavenward in an attitude of prayer,
And unite more intimately with our parents who live up there.

Parents are our earliest teachers, we know,
And always it is sad when we must let them go
In January God's arms reached down, Tony's mom to lift,
And Judith rang the doorbell with her thoughtful gift.

It was a mini-rosebush with 3 blooms of white,
Representing "Besta," Helen, and Marie and their efforts to teach us right.
They did the best they could do and loved us in so many ways
We'll do well to model them as we progress through all our days.

Winter has turned to Spring, the sun is brightly shone,
And we truly rejoice that Judith's breast cancer is gone.
Again there is a gift from Judith, a bright yellow tulip of spring—
And bright jelly beans of joy, like the sparkle surprises God plans to bring.

We know how much He loves us, this is clear,
In the families and friends He's given us so loving and so dear.
He's made the earth His garden, its colorful carpet never ends—
He's even provided the flowers for friends to gift to friends.

Judith and Matt, I thank you for sharing God's bounty
And helping us always to keep aware
Of the Gift of Life laid out for us,
And the friendship that we share.

Early 2001

ONCE UPON A NURSE

*Mimi became special friends with many of the nurses at CBCC in
Bakersfield, where she received her treatment. This is a story
about just one of those nurses, but it could be about any of them.*

Arla is a professional nurse whom I have observed in action.
Many days she begins work before I've even begun to think about a
new day dawning. She is youthful , exciting, and often entertaining to
watch. I hear her relate stories of her life, and I know first-hand that she
is willing to listen to yours when time permits. Her teenage children,
I have learned, are talented and motivated as well as respectful and
sometimes rebellious. She is just as likely to burst at the seams describ-
ing her pride in them as she is to groan in frustration at their latest
foolishness. I guess that's why I like her. She's real.

For Arla being "real" includes wearing what you want to work.
She stays well within professional confines, but picks wild materials for
her smock tops and pays a tailor to create a colorful, working wardrobe
for her. Her hair may be spiked, curly, or teased slightly bouffant, and
in varied hues of orange, blonde, or brunette depending on what suits
her fancy that week. I think she has various colors of contact lenses, too,
because her smiling eyes stand out differently on different days.

Arla has a disciplined assertiveness when circumstances require
compliance. She possesses deep appreciation for the feelings of others,
and uses her spunky sense of humor and spirited sarcastic wit sometimes to soften the seriousness of a situation. Her sense of perspective
serves to establish her as a tolerant caregiver.

This tolerance becomes evident in the things she does as a routine part of her life. On one weekend off, she chaperoned her daughter's softball team over at Pismo Beach for a weekend of friendship
and team bonding activity. She wanted them to learn that when you
work hard, you are also entitled to play hard and have fun. Arla has
the energy to enjoy a bunch of teenage girls, but more importantly, she
wants to teach these kids about simple, satisfying rewards, like leisure
time in their high school world where achievement stresses can sometimes destroy a soul.

When the weekend is over, she comes back to work on Monday

morning, sleep deprived perhaps, but ready for the task at hand. Arla is an oncology nurse in a cancer center.

Today my chart was assigned to her rotation so she had the duty of explaining to me the possible side effects of the new chemo-therapy drug I would be starting. That must be a hard task. She has to appear nonchalant, yet knowledgeable in order to allay unwarranted patient fears while at the same time gaining their confidence and trust in her ability to monitor care. Then she has to poke needles in veins and still maintain your confidence and trust! She has to get the intravenous drip going at the prescribed rate and keep constantly alert for any side effects that might occur.

Alertness is essential for any nurse in this field of work, and her years of mothering her children have served her well. She needs those extra sets of eyes and ears that mothers develop. Arla has developed those eyes in the back of her head. Those eyes that allow you to see what is going on when your back is turned, and she has those ears that can hear warning noises when it is too quiet in a room, three doors down the hall. At work, Arla has to remain attentive to several patients at any given time.

I noticed her casting a glance in my direction to assure that I was doing well, while at the same time she discontinued another patient's IV and sent him home. A while later, she greeted a former patient with warm congratulations when that patient came back to say she was in remission and wanted to share the good news with a nurse who under-stood that special joy. She wandered the room checking her patients and gently covered an elderly, softly snoring man with a light blanket to protect him from the chill of the air-conditioning vent. Moments later, Arla charged out of the room to get extra medication for a young woman affected by sudden-onset anxiety, which many new patients seem to experience. When things were under control, the nurse and patient sat down to discuss the physiological reason for such reactions. The patient was reassured and felt that next time she could remain calmer.

An aura of calmness now seemed to pervade the entire room. Arla took a seat at her central desk to return a phone call concerning a patient at home. After she hung up, she cast a glance toward her two new patients and answered a question for the young woman who had been shaken and scared earlier in the afternoon. It was nice to see this woman smile courageously after their conversation. Next, Arla walked over to the other corner of the room and shared a joke with two fat ladies, dressed alike in red outfits. This pair had been silently chatting together in the corner chairs much of the afternoon. They amused me as they shoved Ritz bits crackers in their mouths and swished them down with Pepsi. One of them had chemotherapy dripping in her arm vein, obviously with no untoward side effects. Her friend had come along to keep her company. It's so amazing to me sometimes that this cancer center can seem so normal. Those happy women dressed in red could have been just as much "at home" in any restaurant in town! I viewed those two ladies in red with admiration at this time. They were feeling fine and having fun. I was winding down from a three-hour intravenous drip and feeling nauseous and very, very tired. Orange, Ritz bits crackers would not have stayed in my stomach for long. Nor did I feel very friendly. I hoped those drops from the intravenous solution ended soon. In a daze, I dozed off momentarily and dreamed that my ride home had arrived and I was out of here.

As I was waking from my short snooze time, I heard someone rustle gently by my chair. I opened my eyes to see Arla sitting again at her desk, charting patient observations and concerns to be addressed by their physicians at a later date. The quiet rustle that had passed my chair was a young girl, about 12 years old, who had come in from the adjacent room and was now approaching Arla at her tall desk. School was over for the day, and this student had come here with her mother who was being treated. I imagine she wanted to lend her mother support and to demonstrate how mature she was in her budding adolescence. Apparently, however, sitting quietly beside her mom in the treatment room became boring for this normally active child. Perhaps the reality of her mom having that dread disease CANCER became apparent as the needle and fluids violated her sweet mother's veins. She had departed from her mother's side in the other room and was looking for somewhere, something.

The girl stopped at Arla's desk and stood next to this nurse with the cool shirt, the spiked hair, and the colored contact lenses.

Hesitatingly, the wandering child asked, " Is there anything I can do here to help you while my mom is resting?"

Experienced, Arla knew how to build confidence as she told the young Miss how, at the end of the day, the pillow cases needed to be changed and freshened up for the next day. The IV poles needed to be rearranged from their random placement around the room and placed neatly beside each recliner chair. The girl looked at the task at hand and appeared to understand. Instructions having been given, Arla thanked the young volunteer and told her how much this assistance would mean at the end of a busy day. Then she poised her pen again and looked down at the stack of charts. The girl didn't move from the desk but had a puzzled look on her face as if she needed further explanation. Arla turned slightly to face the girl and opened her mouth to ask.

Suddenly tears formed in the child's eyes, her face flushed, her bottom lip began to quiver and she cried, "Why does it have to be like this? Why is my mom sick? Is she going to get better? I don't know how to help her!"

Down went Arla's pen, as charts were pushed aside. Pillow cases and poles could wait. Arla stood up and embraced the frightened girl, hugged her tenderly, and let her sob far away from where her mother could see her.

Now tears were rolling down my face too. I felt sadness for the child. I felt thankfulness for the nurse. I hoped that when my own child needs to cry that she will find a shoulder upon which to lay her head, and that there will be someone like Arla there to understand.

CHAPTER 11

Encouragement

FOR MIMI

I called her my "diamond polisher."
She took my written words
Held them in her hands
Softly blew them into clarity
Gently wiped away specks of indistinct meaning.
The ordinary became extraordinary
A diamond in the rough now one of brilliance.

She was a "diamond polisher" friend
She took the people that she knew and loved
Held them in her heart
Softly blew

        Hope for despair
        Faith for doubt
        Joy in sorrow
        Courage in suffering
        Laughter for tears

Gently wiped away specks that clouded vision
The ordinary became extraordinary
The diamond of our lives took on new brilliance.

We now reflect the gifts she gave us
Each of us "polished" in her unique way
May we become "diamond polishers"
Our ongoing gift to her!

Marcia L. Monsma
Friend
February 13, 2004, written for Mimi's memorial service

Feb. 1996

SUPERMAN

When Mimi saw something inspirational, she liked sharing it with others.

2/22/96

Dear Katie,

I hope things are going well in your life. I was thinking of you last night as I was watching Larry King Live! I don't usually watch it, but an advertisement for his show caught my eye . . . so I tuned in.

The guest star was Christopher Reeves, the man who played Superman in the movies. Remember when he was thrown from his horse last year and suffered a spinal cord injury that left him paralyzed from the neck down and dependent on a ventilator to breathe?

I thought his interview was pretty inspirational, and so I'm sharing it with you. For a guy who used to be able to "leap tall buildings in a single bound" it must be very difficult to be confined now to a wheelchair and totally dependent on other people and machines for his existence. What impressed me is that he seems happy and very accepting of his situation. He is striving to overcome his condition and to create a new life doing the things that he is able to do.

Christopher talks about possibly directing movies in the future. He has already begun to write his autobiography, and he hopes to line up speaking engagements to inspire other people and to encourage politicians to put more money into medical research. He is definitely a man with a motive. That, I believe, is the secret to success. We can all use a healthy dose of that!

In the interview, Larry King asked Christopher Reeves if he ever felt sorry for himself and hoped to die. He said there was a short time when he discovered he was paralyzed that he thought death was the easy way out. He felt he would be too big a burden for his family and friends, and he did not want that.

His wife was cool then—she told him that she did not love him only for the things he could do but for whom he was, and she said something along the lines of *YOU are still the same YOU and I love you as much as ever.* That feeling of being unconditionally loved is what gave him the courage to go on living and feeling like a valuable human being. God's love is like that. So is my love for you. Thank you for loving me the same way. I've felt it ever since the beginning. It makes it easy to go through the treatments I have to put up with.

One other statement Reeves made was that the cards and letters of support gave him the incentive to fight to survive and achieve to the best of his ability. I hope that you feel that same encouragement and see the gifts that God gives each day—the sunshine, your family, your friends, the flowers, the inspirations that sometimes just flow through our minds, the music, satisfaction with yourself, your intelligence , creativity, and sense of humor, your fun new dresses, feelings of love and caring . . . the list is endless.

Think about what's good in your life . . . and remember Christopher Reeves. He is a greater hero now than he was as Superman.

Sincerely,

Sept. 1997

POSITIVE THINKING

Mimi was always finding inspirational books to send to other people.

Thursday, September 18, 1997

Dear Mom,

    I am sitting here at the computer doing my book writing. I need a break, and I was just thinking about you so I will type a letter to you. I am feeling gross because I had chemo yesterday. I do not have the energy or incentive to get out. I guess that made me think about how you have been feeling, and I felt sorry for you.

    Unfortunately, feeling sorry for you doesn't make you get any better so I quit feeling sorry, and I decided to do something positive for you instead of sitting here worrying and moping about. I went out to buy you a little cheer-you-up present. I didn't know what to buy. I thought about flowers and figured that, though they are nice, they would die soon, so I didn't send them. I thought about stationery, but you don't write that much. I thought about stitchery you could do to occupy your hands, but I don't think you did the glass case I sent you yet. You said you don't read because your eyes bother you, so I found the perfect choice. A book with large print should not be hard to read. You have a good mind left, and you need to use it.

    I chose a book with thought-provoking and inspirational reading. Each story is short, so you can just read one each day if you wish. BUT I DO WANT YOU TO READ THEM—I may even call and quiz you on them (ha-ha). I have read each one. Some are more meaningful to me than others are, but each one tells of someone's personal thoughts or experiences. Some made me laugh and some made me cry, but every one of them made me think of someone besides myself.

    I find that when I am thinking of someone else, it is next to impossible to feel sorry for myself or worry about things that I have no control over. I give all my worrying to God—He made me, He loves me, He knows what is best for me . . . and besides He is much bigger than me. I like letting Him be in control of my life. The stories in this book are mostly about people who willingly accept the will of God in their lives. Page 40 is a good, short one that all of us could stand to say everyday. No one on this earth (including Jesus Himself) gets through life without trials and suffering. We have to learn to take our suffering and "offer it up" as you often said to me when I was a little girl. I must have listened, and I thank you for the lesson, because I usually am pretty good at it now.

Hope you find value in this book. Share the thoughts you find in it with your friends. It will give you something new to talk about.

Feb. 1996

FAITHFULNESS

Mimi gave encouragement to all of her friends.

Dear Pat,

Happy Valentine's!!! I talked to Betty last night and was really happy to hear that John has good reports from the new drug. Last time I talked to you, he had just begun it and was thinking he had some stomach trouble because of it. He hadn't yet reached full dose yet. I knew you all could do it!!! Stomach aches are a little easier to take when you know that they are producing good results elsewhere.

I hear that the prolactin levels have dropped way down, and that indeed is encouraging news. It sounds like John falls into the category of the one-third that responds well to this new drug. I felt certain he would.

You know, Pat, when you think about John—well, why shouldn't he be in that blessed third???? How many kids are #1 in the eighth grade? One out of a hundred?????? If he can pull off that feat and be 1 in a class of 100, then it just makes sense that he could easily be in the top third of good responders to this new drug. He's just a remarkable kid all around!!!

We have him in our prayers out here, and I am certain that prayer blows the winds of change in a direction most beneficial to us.

I'm sorry if he is having stomach and intestinal problems—unfortunately, it is one of the downsides of this heavy-duty medicine. A few secrets I've learned about good nutrition—it is VERY IMPORTANT to keep it up even if you don't feel like eating.

It's easy to turn healthy food into good tasting shakes by mixing them in the blender. Fruit smoothies go down really easily—use sherbet or flavored yogurt, fruit juice or milk, vanilla ice cream, and any kind of fruit you can get your hands on—ripe bananas, canned peaches, pears, pineapple, strawberries, and applesauce.

Puddings are good to coat your stomach, and don't overlook some of those good baby food desserts—custards, etc. Also, if he can't swallow vitamins some days, try baby squirt Poly Vi Sol, etc. (You can mix it in the fruit smoothies.) Lots of high energy liquid nutrition drinks are on the market in many different flavors—Ensure is pretty good, as is Boost. Malt-O-Meal, mashed potatoes, whipped Jell-O with cream cheese and fruit added—all add good nutrition and variety without too much need for heavy digestion when your stomach is acting up.

At the rate John should be growing now, with the restart of growth hormone, he needs to be sure to eat plenty of good food. We want to keep that young man growing strong!!!!

I'm doing very well. As I told Betty, I finally feel like I am working my way back into the mainstream of society. I still have some restrictions the weeks I'm on chemotherapy. I have to avoid crowds, but I have found meaningful small group activities—babysitting for my friend's triplets (with their mom, of course), my Christian Writer's Critique workshop, and lunches, always lunches . . . and my waistline and derrière attest to that. I'm so mad about the size they are becoming, BUT I LOVE MY INNER SELF!!! (How's that for a secure attitude??)

Anyhow, I told Betty I would mail her my latest idea for a chapter in my book. I am very proud of it. I still think it's funny, and I'm especially happy I found the FOR BETTER OR WORSE COMIC STRIP. I have an extra copy, so I'm sending one to you too. If you see Kay or Jeren, you can share it with them, but I thought you and Betty would appreciate it most.

Also, Pat, I have begun the reflections of Moses, but I am finding a hard time finishing up. I do intend to finish this for you and for myself. I enjoy doing it . . . but since it will take you a while to read it, I'll just send the beginning now. The rest will arrive in installments . . .

NEVER GIVE UP!!! CELEBRATE THE GOOD NEWS!!!! ACKNOWLEDGE THE FATHER (HE created John and knows every inch of him like no one else—John is just exactly who the Father created him to be). Intercede to the SON (He understands suffering and the weak human condition). Listen to the HOLY SPIRIT (He was Jesus' parting gift to His people after His ascension into Heaven and He knows our hearts) . . . Hold on to the good test results and the days of high spirits—they can buoy you up on the bleaker days (which we pray will be few).

I've got to run along , Pat, if I hope to get this in the mail today.

Keep your spirits up. Remember to pray for John's doctors always—that they will have wisdom, discernment, and understanding. God is using their research and their knowledge and their dedication along with your FAITHFULNESS to produce great things. As the man born blind, I think John is being used so that the works of God might be made manifest in him (John 9:3). Your family has always and is currently doing a beautiful job of this. Keep up the good work!

Oct. 2000

HEALING

*Mimi would always talk to the person sitting next to her at chemo.
She met many new friends that way.*

October 2, 2000

Dear Mary,

You have been in my thoughts and prayers since I met you last week at CBCC. It was inspiring to me to talk with you and Mark and to witness your positive attitude and courage. I hope you have survived the initial "yuk" days following chemotherapy with minimal discomfort and frustration. I thought of you often as I am very empathetic to that toxic, nauseated, fatigued, drugged, confusion state that our bodies go through in their recovery process. Obnoxious, isn't it?

Think of it this way, Mary—if the strong cells in your body reacted the way they did to that chemotherapy, just imagine what that medicine was able to do to those unfriendly cancer cells. That chemo is strong stuff, no doubt about it—but remember, You are even stronger . . . because we have the power of God behind us.

I do hope you can feel God's healing touch at work in your body, and that you will vow to be kind to yourself. Your body has been through so much—the emotional shock, the surgery, the chemotherapy. Rest is so important. Your good white and red blood cells need time to build themselves up and recover—it's like getting over the flu, it takes time to gain strength. Cancer teaches us patient endurance. Embrace the peaceful, reflective times, and enjoy quiet moments together with your family. Life will return to its wild, fast-moving pace again next year . . . and you will be ready . . . and running !

Nov. 1997

KEEP IT UP

Mimi always took time to care for her mom.

Dear Mom,

It was so nice to talk to you Friday night. Your voice sounded so much stronger, and I can tell that you are benefiting from your classes at the hospital. I have found that talking about difficult things helps me to cope with life better. My psychologist, Corey, has been through many of the same things I have been through. He had cancer when he was 22. Now he is 32 and is perfectly healthy. He is healthy in his body and in his mind. He has talked out and worked through his anxieties and fears. He has developed a deep spirituality. He says he still gets worried about things—financial worries, recurrence of his cancer, worry about his parents' health, concern that he is being a good husband for his cute wife, concern that he may not be able to have his own biological child because chemotherapy ten years ago may have destroyed his ability to produce sperm, etc.

He knows that worries are normal, but he does not allow them to diminish his enthusiasm and joy for life. I told him that I feel that way too. I cannot control most of the things I worry about—so I try to cast off the worries and enjoy life. Corey and I both realize that we have survived cancer and when we look back at that experience we see that although it was hard, we were strong enough to overcome it. We came to realize through the experience how precious and valuable life is—and we intend to live life to the fullest and to use our strength and knowledge to help others. It is evident to both of us that God intended that we should remain on this earth, and we are forever grateful for such a loving God. We know we can turn to Him when worries and anxieties get us down.

Mom, you have gone through some rough experiences, especially recently. You survived brain surgery, a ruptured appendix, and panic anxiety, which left you hospitalized. It takes energy and determination, understanding, attention, and a lot of hard work to improve. I know you never were a great student in school, but it sounds like you are paying attention to these new psychology lessons you are learning in therapy. These are important lessons. Keep up the good work. I am proud of you.

I talked to Kathy Davy yesterday. I wanted to find out how her mother is doing after her brain aneurysm. She is very tired but seems to be doing well. I'm glad for that. Kathy told me she is planning to have Thanksgiving and is looking forward to having everybody together. Your potato salad and vegetable dish sound like they will be really good additions to Thanksgiving Dinner. I'm glad you will be feeling well enough to go.

I hope your therapy sessions continue to go well at the hospital.

Remember—improving at anything is hard work. Keep at it.

CHAPTER 12

Other Stories

I first heard of Mimi through a mutual friend, Mary. Mimi and Mary both were at the baptism of my 3-month-old triplets during 10:30 Mass at St. Philip the Apostle Church.

During the Mass that morning, Msgr. Ronald Swett, who baptized my babies, had mentioned to the assembly to let Cindy know if there was anyone who could come to the house to help with them. Within a day or so, Mary called me and said that she had a friend who was at the baptism that wanted to come help and so did her oldest daughter, Christine. Mary gave me a brief insight about them. She said that Mimi had been battling cancer but was doing well and that she was a wonderful person. She said that Mimi's daughter, Christine, had just finished medical school and was in a residency program at Kern Medical Center here in Bakersfield.

Me, being the over-protective Mom that I had fast become, trusted in our mutual friend Mary's opinion and let the "strangers" in my house. First came Christine. I could tell she instantly fell in love with being around babies. She even shared her dreams of someday having children of her own and would welcome the idea of twins!!! A week or so later, I met Mimi at a 7:00 A.M. Mass. (Brad, my husband, and I were going to separate Masses at the time for obvious reasons). Mimi introduced herself to me after Mass. I was so glad to put a face with her name after all I had come to learn about her from her daughter. She seemed so pleasant and displayed such a warm spirit about her that I just knew she would be "OK" to let in my house.

The day came when Mimi made it over to my house. That was the beginning of a wonderful journey with an unexpected, special friend, who I bonded with in such a short amount of time. She always had a pleasant smile and positive attitude. She had more energy than I did. She loved to play with my kids and teach them The *Wheels On the Bus* song even before they could sit up on their own. She was the first person to spontaneously offer to sit with the babies so Brad and I could go out for Valentine's Day!

Brad and I forgot what we used to talk about and didn't quite know what to do with ourselves that evening, but we did appreciate the kindness of a new found, fast friend who obviously knew what it was like to be a parent.

Mimi became a fairly regular visitor at our house. She usually came when she was in-between chemo treatments and her immune system was fairly strong. She shared a lot about her journey with cancer as we played with and fed the babies. On her "good days," even if she was wearing a "port-a-cath" in her chest and carrying a chemo pump like you would a purse, she would say to me, "Let's take the kids on a field trip." I was so ready to get out of the house with an extra set of hands that I had no problem taking her up on her offer!

Needless to say, Mimi became part of our lives. Little did I know that God would send me a person to support me in the issues I had regarding one of my babies having motor skill problems; little did I know that the things she shared with me about cancer would apply to my dad who was diagnosed for the first time when the babies were almost 2 years old; little did I know that she would become involved in the RCIA ministry that Brad and I have been involved in since 1991 and that she would sponsor a very special, young, lady doctor that had issues with her mother passing away from cancer and was angry inside (what a major witness to Brad and I and others, especially the young lady doctor); little did I know that she would be instrumental in getting to know my dad during his chemo treatments and providing him with a surely "God-given" peace for his own cancer journey; little did I know that she and her youngest daughter, Liz, would participate in Dad's funeral by bring up "the gifts" (in my mind, it was symbolic of the necessary gift they gave to my dad during chemo treatments);

Five months later, Mimi went home too! The only way my dad was able to participate in her funeral was with his collection of Irish CD's. He just happened to have the song *When Irish Eyes Are Smiling*, which I copied and wrote down the words for some of Mimi's musical, Irish family to sing at her graveside service.

A few weeks before her departure, I was able to visit her. I didn't expect to . . . but I was so glad when Liz met me at the car as I was delivering a meal, a card, and some flowers. I was so glad that it was all right for the kids to come visit her too. I knew they needed to, and I felt that Mimi needed to see them one last time as well. Mimi was so frail (seemed like all of a sudden). She was obviously in pain and having difficulty breathing (she was hooked up to oxygen and heavily medicated for pain), but she was still smiling and obviously not wanting to worry us or make us think she wasn't doing well. I think she somehow realized that she wasn't fooling us (as sweet as it was of her), and in her own way, said her good-bye to us. I tried so hard to keep a straight face for this woman who was at all my kid's birthdays and even their First Holy Communion. Her faith was very important to her. She recognized the demands and pleasures of being a mom. She was a good mother to her own four children. She realized the important job of being a wife and trying to juggle that with trying to find and keep your own identity. She realized the importance of friendship and community.

Mimi was so much a part of our lives that my children wanted to know "what she was to us" (how she was related) when she died. Mimi will always live in our hearts, as I'm sure she is living in the hearts of many others.

Cindy Webb
Friend

Jan. 1996

Mimi wrote many letters to Dr. Patel over the years. Here is just one.

January 20, 1996

Dear Dr. Patel,

I'm sitting here at my computer and trying different things. I am beginning to have some mastery over this machine. It feels pretty good. I'm reporting back to you on my experience so far with that new prescription, Melatonin. Yes, it is over the counter. The first night I took it was very strange. Falling asleep, I felt like I was getting seasick, with the sensation of being on a ship going up and down. My head and stomach didn't feel very good, but at the same time my joints and limbs felt very warm and TOTALLY relaxed. It was easy to fall asleep.

That drug did the same thing as Tylenol PM. It put me to sleep quickly and very soundly . . . for about three hours. Then I was wide awake, supercharged, very hot, and could not settle down for two to three hours. When I finally did drop back to sleep again, it was very deep . . . and then it was hard to get up with Tony's alarm at 6:00 the next morning. That's the kind of sleeping pattern Sue Helper doesn't like. She says my neurological system really needs a more solid stretch of sleeping. The same thing happened the next night. On the third night, I decided not to take any Melatonin . . . and I slept for six hours straight through.

Last night I was up late and was not feeling at all tired, but it was after midnight so I figured I should get to bed. I took another of those tablets so I could fall asleep, which I did immediately, and I slept straight through for 6 or 7 hours . . . so I guess my body is beginning to get used to them. I think it will work.

Also I hope Dr. Bhogal's office sent you a copy of the colonoscopy and biopsy report. I asked them to do so. Apparently, it was sent only to Sue Helper's office since she was the original referral name on the top of the chart. Also, I was supposed to have scheduled an appointment with Dr. Bhogal two weeks after the exam so he could discuss the results with us. I did not remember being told that so I never went. It's not smart to tell people those things after the "space-out" drugs they use for that procedure. You don't remember much. Oh, well.

I am typing my book. My major critics here (Tony and the girls) say it is too "church-y," and I need to add some humor. I'm sure that will cause it to have more appeal. The ability to laugh is vital in a crisis situation. You know that. Actually, I thought this wig story part was pretty funny and so did they. So I figured I would send you a copy because you deal all day long with serious problems, and I just want you to know there is a lighter side too.

I'm getting more disciplined. I have joined a Writer's workshop where we critique one another's works. Several of the ladies in my group have published manuscripts already, and so they know the Writer's market and are willing to share their knowledge. I think this will work out well, but this is a much harder project than I thought. One good thing is that I found someone who will help me type. I met Patty Duke, one of Shawn's patients with colon cancer, who is an executive secretary. Now I just have to figure out the best way to get what is in my brain out through her much more efficient (than mine) typing fingers . . . oh, life is full of challenges . . .

Have a good day

June 2001

Mimi felt it important, once in a while, to thank her doctors
for everything they do.

June 21, 2001

Dear Dr. Patel,

Thank you for your attentiveness when I met with you two weeks ago. Despite your busy schedule, I once again left your office knowing that you carefully listened. Thank you for the positive affirmations you offered.

I, too, am very happy that the CEA roller coaster ride prior to, during, and immediately after radiation has begun to head down. I hope it continues to hit ground level. If it doesn't go down there where it's supposed to, I figure I might be a good candidate for the new drug . . . after it goes through the final phase of controlled studies. I'm happy to let other people test it out first. I'd like not to need it.

Right now, I feel like I'm doing fine on the 5-FU pump. Thank you for your concern that it might be "too inconvenient" for me. Actually it has become like an appendage, and it's not all that hard to handle . . . except for the side effects at the end of the cycle. I appreciate how you carefully listened as I tried to ask if there was a better way of scheduling treatment to avoid side effects like skin blistering, muscle and joint stiffness, and low white counts.

That was a hard question to deliver because I know that those inconvenient side effects typically accompany 5-FU. I know I can and will tolerate them. However, I also have considered lately that there must be a way to improve on the body-depleting side effects while still maintaining adequate control of the cancer growth. Thank you for allowing me to explain my rationale, and even asking me to repeat my question when I didn't easily convey my thinking process the first time. I know you listened carefully, respected my ideas, and were willing to try a different treatment schedule. A trial period of 20 days on/10 days off until mid-August sounded very appealing to me. With a current CEA of 6, I feel we have some leeway to try a less harsh dosing schedule. I also am resigned to the reality that at this time I have to remain on some form of chemotherapy.

I was especially happy, however, that we agreed to delay for five days the initiation of my being hooked up to the pump again. I just wasn't ready. By Monday I was mentally and physically prepared to begin again, and I noted that the wimpy total of white cells and granulocytes were up from the appointment day five days before. Though it may be purely psychological, I just felt stronger on Monday than I had on Wednesday. I have since learned that my CEA went up from 5.8 to 6.0 during the twelve days that I was off the pump. That may be a statistically insignificant change, but it provides the evidence I need to know I still can't slack off . . . and I won't.

I know you are aware of and value the motivation I have to be successful in coping with my cancer. I have been blessed with strong faith, a supportive family, progress, success, and caring friends. I also have been most fortunate to have an oncologist who listens, encourages, and sends me off always with something to think about. The thought I took from your last visit was your quote, "I think of what I do as more ART than science." I have come to know and appreciate that this is true of you. The way you patiently weave your knowledge of science respectfully with the physical, mental, emotional, and spiritual needs of your patients is truly an art. Science is knowledge and intelligence; Art is Wisdom.

Everyone knows you are intelligent. Thank you for being wise.

March 1998

Another letter to Dr. Patel.

March 18, 1998

Dear Dr. Patel,

Thank you for calling Monday night—not so much for the information you conveyed—but for being so attentive. I appreciate the fact that you allowed me to go on alternate weeks for the past eight months. I needed the break from the intensity of weekly treatments. That amount of time also allowed me to come to the same conclusion that you did, namely, alternate weeks was not working as the most effective solution to my problem.

I know I can do EVERY week—I've done it before. I don't like it, but sometimes we just have to do things we don't like. I'll just go to matinees at Edwards Cinema (relaxing activity) instead of cleaning the house and making dinner(supreme stress)—I'll be happy doing that as my way of coping, though you'll probably have to start treating Tony for spousal frustration! I'm just kidding, of course, but I thought that sounded like a pretty funny idea . . . and I know I must maintain my sense of humor.

Actually, your decision came at a good time. I had finally started to learn to ignore my CEA's and go on with a positive approach to life, taking one day at a time and not jumping ahead to the future over which I have little control. I've had some incredible opportunities over the past couple months, occasions which just seemed to force me to focus on the value of my life and the lessons I've learned through my trials.

I've attended a writing and speaking seminar in Fresno, a retreat/ mission at our church (Topic: Compassion and Going Within to the Heart), read most of Bernie Siegel's latest book, worked out various minor problems with Corey Gonzales' aid, and was able to encourage several other cancer survivors during crises periods in their lives.

One of the advantages I see of speaking to other survivors is that the positive information I try to convey to them becomes more entrenched in my own way of thinking. The effort is well worth it, but I'm taking that slow because I've learned that this type of support group and individual counseling can become overwhelming. I am, however, being greatly encouraged by my Bible Study this year. We are studying about Paul, the evangelist and disciple of Christ. His letters, which are in the Bible, are beautiful and worthy guides to living.

Just before you called Monday evening, I had returned from a lecture and discussion where I learned that Paul wrote many of these letters while he was in prison for his "radical" teaching. He was chained to a prison guard, yet he completed some of his finest work. I'll use Paul as my own object lesson; chained to IV chemotherapy, I'll aim to do the same.

Have a good day. Actually, have many good days. I will see you at the end of April when I return from my short trip to San Antonio. Then you can tell me my CEA is dropping!

Sincerely,

Jan. 1998

SECURITY

Even in her weariness, Mimi was always thinking about other people.

It is in helping others that we usually help ourselves. I think I heard it first from my mother, and I have had it proven over and over and over again in my life . . . but I forget it so easily. For several months now, I have been preoccupied with my own problems. In August, it was the promise of weaning off chemotherapy and the resultant fear that weaning wouldn't work. In November it was the reality that "I wouldn't be weaned by Christmas." By December that reality had turned again. "Will I ever be off? Will I ever be Free? Will I ever get organized? How long will I have to go on with a good week/a bad week/a good week/ a bad week, etc. etc.

Christmas seemed to highlight my problem. I decided to keep my nose to the grindstone, to bite the bullet as they say. I got things done—bought gifts, shopped the sales with Christine, mailed out of town packages, went to the parties, made some cookies, shuffled the kids in and out, made beds, greeted house guests, cooked, cleaned, put up the Christmas tree, and took down the Christmas tree. I did the things, but I sacrificed quality time with the people I love to be with. We got lots of Christmas cards, but I didn't write a one. It's January 10 and that still bugs me . . .

One of the victories of the holiday season is that I think I succeeded in reestablishing that I am the female head of this household. That seemed like something I needed and wanted to do. Apparently, I did it very convincingly by being able to do alternate week chemo and still accomplish all that was needed in the way of hospitable hostess and daily and nightly mom. The kids relaxed at Thanksgiving and Christmastime, and they went off on ski trips, to Vegas, and to the movies. It made me feel good. I like to see them free and happy and independent, but as Julie Davy said, "her mom is jealous of the exciting single life." Though I would never choose to go back to that age group, and though I would never change any of the circumstances of my life, I am envious of the stages in life and the relative security that our children have . . .

Maybe that is the point. They have that security and I don't. I've been prone to pity parties lately and that makes me angry. I know how much I have to be thankful for. I don't like to allow those pity parties, but it seems I have had a lot of down time, and I've let my head fill up with thoughts that get me off balance (CEA counts, the future, insurance, my mom, the relationship of my siblings, Tony's dad, and all his family, Tony's health, and his job security). I'm trying to prioritize my days: exercise with Deborah, Mass, school, writing, volunteering, taking time to help friends. Short-term I want to help Cindy teach the kids, help Judith through back surgery, and help Heidi get the volunteer program restarted at Hoffmann. I want to remain in Bible Study, keep at least minimally involved with the Cancer Society, figure out ways to spend quality time with Tony, sympathize with Christine and the stresses of work and job hunt, and write occasionally to the kids and encourage them. I want to sit back each day and GAIN PERSPECTIVE.

I have lots on the back burner—reading, movies, visualization therapy.

I have not been able to sort out much of anything the past several weeks. Christmas ended; the house got quiet . . . I had a couple good days and felt like I was getting it together. Then I had chemo, then I got the flu, then I had chemo again before I was fully recovered, now scans loom on the horizon, and then I wait for my appointment with Dr. Patel where we discuss our next plan of attack. I am weary of being sick.

Mid-2000

GOD'S GUIDE

*This story tells of Mimi's entrance into the lives of the Webb family
who went on to become very special family friends.*

In the Meantime . . .

I spent the first 25 years of my marriage anticipating children, having children, working and playing with children, or teaching, disciplining, and raising children. That was my job. Although there were times I was exhausted, times I was bored, times I feared I was becoming brain-dead, times I was frightened, times I was challenged, times I was deflated, and times I was overwhelmed . . . I must say that I loved those years!

Now my home is void of the voices of children, teenagers, and young adults. I'm in an empty nest. Our young adults are on their own and discovering the challenges that await them in this new millennium. They are directed in their career paths, perhaps searching for spouses, and walking upon a path largely unknown to me . . .

That twenty-fifth year of our marriage provided my children with probably the most difficult final exam they would ever take. Their world of childhood was tested with the challenge that would compel them to put into practice all that they had learned. They had to allay my fears, ease my anxiety, renew my confidence, and give me the courage to go on. They had to convince me that Love was more powerful than any inconvenience I had caused them.

I never doubted for a moment that God had given us exceptional children. I just never realized how exceptional . . .

(unity, friendships, sacrifices, patience, joy)

Where God guides He provides . . .

Useful . . . I needed a job. That's what I needed once again. Any experience??? Twenty-five years of raising a family. Any limitations? Not much energy.

Go to Mass on the Baptismal day of the Webb triplets. I love ceremonies in the church. Mass. Baptisms. First Holy Communions. Confirmations. Weddings. Even A couple Holy Orders. I like the processions. This one was especially appealing to me because there were babies in it. I wanted to reach out and touch someone . . .

I did a couple Sundays later when I saw Cindy at 7:00 Sunday Mass, and I asked her if she would like my help sometime. She was quiet and graceful. I liked her. I think she trusted me to help her hold and feed her babies.

She was wise and encouraging. She showed perfect understanding and patience with my needs. And the kids . . .

Well, they have provided a measuring stick for me. Sometimes I feel that I have accomplished little in the past five years. The stagnation I feel makes me sad. Then I have a day like yesterday when the kids come over and they swim . . . and we laugh and play and I realize what five years means.

The triplet's birth was a miracle. Each life is a miracle. Each occurrence in each life is a miracle.

Zach is a cautious little boy. He thinks before he acts, and he thinks before he talks. He shows great consideration for people's feelings. He wanted to follow Riley when he saw how much fun Riley had jumping off the diving board. He proceeded to the board, stood gingerly upon it, and looked at the high distance between the end of the board and the water below. The Deep end. Then he took a careful step backward and stepped cautiously back down to the deck of the pool. Saving face, he explained to those who were watching, " I don't want to jump off the diving board; I'm afraid I might break it!" One who knows Zach well knows that he cares for all "living" things . . . even diving boards!

So he returned to the shallow water where he gradually became brave enough to jump off the top step into the shallow water. Height was not important here. Speed was. He worked up speed as he whirled his arms around him, gathering momentum with each new movement. Garnering courage in this way, he would eventually jump into my waiting arms, held out to him at "just the right" jumping distance. Adding decorum to his feat of bravery, he called his jump "my super speeder." He flapped and wound his arms up furiously before the jump. The sense of power was reflected on his face, the feeling of security was certain because all these preliminaries were conducted on safe dry land . . . and then came the tentative jump. Success. No water in the nose. No drowning. The catching arms held tight. Fun! We'll try it again. This time more boldly. Do it again. And again. And again. The Super Speeder was established, and Zach was feeling really good about the whole process. Climbing to the top step, as he got ready to begin another "Super Speeder" wind-up, high on life as a little child gets, he turned to me and said with a communal bond of Love, "God gives me the power to do these Super Speeders."

Like I said, if you know Zach, you know how much he cares for all living things. He Knows God is alive . . .

PERSPECTIVES

Mimi was able to see a lesson in everything she did.

"What did you do today?" someone asked.

I answered, "Well, I had fun watching little 2-year-old triplets figure out how to climb up a ladder to go down the slide."

"Sounds fun," was the slightly sarcastic answer I received.

I replied, "As a matter of fact, it was not only fun, but exciting, exhausting, and very educational."

It was exciting especially from the point of view of the 2-year-olds. This was a new skill to be tackled, an adventure just waiting to happen. The reward was great; they got to stand up in the log fort atop the ladder and look down to the ground and see what it looked like from a seven-foot perch. They were BIG and mom-standing-on-the-ground was little. How important they must have felt . . . and how proud was mom! There was some initial trepidation at the top of the slide while looking down, but MOMMY was at the bottom of the slide with her arms outstretched to catch them. As fun as it was at the top of the world, there was nothing that could compare to the feel of mom's arms. So down they went eagerly.

It was exhausting because the 2-year-olds wanted to try it again . . . and again. . . . and again. As Mommy's arms ached from reaching up to assist them on the ladder and my arms ached from reaching down to pull them up to the platform, the little ones' eager faces would line up ready to "do it again." Their zest for living and their joy at trying new skills makes even the most energetic adult feel somewhat envious.

It was educational because they learned new skills that day. It was hard work as they reached their little legs about as far as they would stretch in order to reach the next higher rung of the ladder. Then while their body hung slightly unbalanced, one hand had to let go for a moment to stretch higher up the ladder post . . . then the other hand . . . then the feet. Repeat. Then sit down at the edge of the platform, slide down, start over. Practice. They'll work up to the expert level someday. Each of them, and they'll work up to continuously bigger challenges as their lives go on.

I was thinking later that day how much the babies lives resemble our own. We are constantly beset by challenges, and we will accomplish them successfully if we can maintain the same level of enthusiasm as those little kids. We will be able to take big steps only by letting go of some of the security pillars in our lives. We need to stop sometimes and take an overview of the world around us(the platform). We need to make decisions (to slide or not to slide). Then we need to be renewed and rewarded and caught up by those we love and trust. Finally, we need to practice . . . again and again and again.

God is ever there to assure us as we climb, to catch us when we slide. All we need to do is trust Him . . . and watch a baby grow in order to know his faithfulness.

Riley, Samantha, and Zach—Grab your mother, and let's go to the park again!

Nov. 1997

FISH HEADS AND RICE

Sometimes, you have to look at the positive side of your deficits. Mimi was thankful on several occasions that she did not have a sense of smell. It was a constant running joke in her family, "Mom how does this smell??"

November 12

Today at chemotherapy the number of nauseated people seemed greater than usual. When I walked in and took my chair, I noticed that most people were speaking and sympathizing with the sick-looking ones next to them. I thought it was just a friendly crowd being nice to the less fortunate ones.

Then Kathy, my nurse, apologized for the bad smell. I didn't smell anything so I figured that it was probably a patient who threw up, and I wasn't going to make a big deal about that. I know only too well that sometimes you can't help it, and in a group environment that can be terribly embarrassing.

I noticed that some of the nurses were laughing at one of the other nurses and sharing some light-hearted "in" joke. It was not like them to be insensitive, especially at a patient's expense. So I asked Kathy what was so funny. She said, "Fish heads. Can't you smell them?"

"Well, no. As a matter of fact, I cannot. That sense went out along with my brain tumor . . . but how did fish heads get in here anyway?" I asked, noticing that some other patients were looking incredulously at me. "I don't smell anything."

Knowing that some of the chemotherapy agents are produced from animal by-products and knowing that shark cartilage is hypothesized to ward off cancer, I thought maybe some unique experimentation was going on in the lab with fish heads. I was being cool about it, not wanting to question any alternative techniques for treatment.

Kathy was trying hard to tend to her more serious nursing duties, but she couldn't help laughing as she told me about her co-worker nurse, Karen. Karen is a gentle, compassionate nurse who noticed that one of her patients had brought along a bite of casserole lunch, which she was eating as she waited in the treatment room. Karen thought it did not look very appetizing eaten cold, so she offered to heat it up for the woman. The woman seemed grateful for the offer and Karen kindly placed it in the microwave. It was in the microwave for a few seconds on full power when . . . Ping! . . . Pong! . . . Karen rushed to retrieve the rice dish before it exploded anymore.

She whipped open the door of the oven. Then a smell wafted through the room and made everyone gag. The casserole was rice and fish heads . . . whose petite, pea-sized eyes could not take the heat and popped right out of their tiny, little, fish heads.

. . . Sometimes I have no regrets that I have lost my ability to smell when offered this type of unique opportunity.

Aug. 1996

SUPPORT GROUPS

*This was a reflection of Mimi's on the necessity of support groups
whether in the traditional sense or not.*

August 30

Today I went to lunch at Olive Garden with Julie Worthing and Mary Lou Sabas. There was some talk about support groups. I GOT TO THINKING ABOUT MINE. Oops! Amparo called and said Vince Perez was talking about starting a support group in our parish; Amparo wants to add healing masses to it—perhaps in a general healing ministry sort of way, perhaps a Cancer Support Group.

My experience with cancer support groups has not been very positive. I went to Jeff Schulman's group for asthmatic children, and there were quite a bunch of whiny mothers there. I didn't have much patience. The dynamics were not well controlled. I went once to Dr. Patel's support group. The people were mostly older, attended regularly, kind of liked it for a night out . . . but I didn't need a night out. I went out all day. The woman that began to smoke as soon as she hit the parking lot turned me agitated immediately. Chris and Katie were with me; they were neutral to negative. Mostly they felt nothing was accomplished, sort of a waste of time.

Vince, being a professional, could probably effectively lead a support group. Next question. Singles or couples, family???

Where are my support groups. When diagnosed with cancer, one is hit head on with the reality of their mortality. I felt alone and numb. My first support came from my family who were just present, reminding me that they cared—then acting normal, laughing in my room, reminding me that life goes on, coping mechanisms, my birthday party reminding me that life is special and can be filled with fun. The nurses and doctors who understood my insecurities—Nancy and the port a cath, Dr. P and his family meeting, Sue Helper and her "I'm sorry," then supporting Dr. P and trusting him, cooperative, even Phillips with his stark honesty.

Mortality fears were assuaged by the group from church, the BSF people. I needed to believe that God knew I was here and that I got to know Him well—I didn't want to go to the home of a stranger.

The Mare group and the way those children and families handled disability. I, too, could deal with mine, colostomy, if necessary, etc. The back brace had been easy with them.

My family all calling from Chicago and all the flowers and cards, even at Christmas. The answers back: I will pray for you, sorry you are sick, Elaine, Adele, Bud—I could always tell him—Lenni, Gram, GrampJen angels, meals from the office.

Betty Kay Pat Joan Hug and visit.

The kids because of their ages and intelligence and love, Chris managing the house long distance, Katie coming home for a year, Liz watching after me, her mother-child, David and his courage and acceptance, manhood. Tony because of his thoroughness and knowing I was getting the best medical care, relief. My mother because she made me cover up because of her weakness. If I died, she would die, and then I would have been responsible for killing my mother. My dad because he taught me how to live patiently and accept infirmity without shame.

The Medical society ladies, Mary Caratan, and the women who helped me through brain recovery. Then the hospice group who by their presence could ease the fear of the process of dying (I felt secure covering all the bases!) and remind me that I would never die alone, and I need not have to suffer or be in a sterile environment.

Those who looked to me for support. Patty Duke in the parking lot, Five feet under, Toni Gallardo, Julie coming to the Cancer Plaza Dedication, Jell Lane, and Darren Oliver and then my secret angels therapeutic, then Belinda Julie Mary Lou. Kathy Davy Dad story-songs.

Books Lenni, Richard Bloch, Ronie Kaye, Writers support group

Julie, Mary Lou, Belinda, me—communication problem with our spouses (Toni G. too) Use Pete and Sheryl as an example. Family scenes can make us sad as we envision ourselves not in them. Our humanness comes out sometimes. We feel worry and guilt, should not allow this. I AM. We will help each other better because of this however (Bible . . . trials).

Mary Lou—earrings and ladies from church praying (Hebrews 1:14).

Eight-year-old. It's ok if you die; Dad will marry and I will like the new mom. With one another, it is easier to talk about our vulnerabilities.

Composine and Kaopectate cocktails

Colonoscopy clean

MIMI DEETHS EULOGY—

By Christine Deeths, M.D.

Good Morning and welcome. It seems almost fitting to gather today on Valentine's Day, a holiday whose symbol is the heart, to celebrate the life of my mother.

When I was in the tenth grade, my English teacher gave us what seemed like a nearly impossible assignment, and she gave us only one week to complete it. She wanted us to write an essay about our heroes. Your heroes, she said, are what define who you are and what is important to you. Heroes are important people like the President or the Mayor. They are movie stars, rock singers, or athletes. Heroes are someone famous that everybody knows.

For most of the week, I struggled with her definition of hero. I could not think of anyone who was worthy of hero status. The day before the assignment was due, I had still not come up with a hero. I sat at home that night utterly frustrated and worried that I would never pass tenth grade English. So I did what all good children do—I went and sniveled to my Daddy. I told him how unfair the assignment was. Then in the matter-of-fact way he seemed to reserve only for his distraught children, he explained to me that my problem was not that I did not have a hero, but rather the teacher had given me an faulty standard of heroism.

Heroes, he said, are people who change your life for the better and have a lasting impact on the world around them. Heroes are people who make a difference. Heroes do not have to be famous. Anyone can be a hero. Heroes, he said, are the people you most want to grow up to be.

I finished my essay that night and passed tenth grade English, but I got a greater gift as well. I realized that night what makes a true hero. As I sat down this week to write a Eulogy for my mother, I was reminded of that essay and that conversation because my mother was and still is one of my heroes.

As a tenth grader, I had a difficult time defining exactly what made my mom a hero, but back then I only had to write an introduction, three paragraphs of five sentences each, and a conclusion. Plus, I only had 15 years worth of experiences to draw from. Today, my task is a little more daunting; partly because it is impossible to sum up someone like my mother in 15 sentences, and partly because I have 18 more years of memories to draw from.

There were so many special things about my mom that narrowing them down and picking just a few seems impossible.

From my earliest memories, my mom was always doing something for someone. At first, I think that someone was usually me, but as Katie, David, and Liz were added to the family, she was able to make us all feel special and loved. She was the best kind of mom, young and vigorous, active and involved, but still had the time to kiss our skinned knees, build forts and villages in the basement, which sometimes to the chagrin of dad, she did not always make us clean up. She nurtured our creativity and curiosity. She let us make mistakes but also helped us learn from them. She and Dad allowed us to know them, love them, laugh with them, and cry with them. The memories of our time together as a family are the most precious to me.

I remember countless family celebrations, holidays, birthdays with cakes made with love and decorations, and gifts picked with care. I remember family vacations with exciting destinations, museums, and tourist attractions carefully chosen by dad with suitcases and treats packed away by mom. I remember family weddings, parties, and reunions at the lake with lots of fun and laughter. I remember hot chocolate with marshmallows on cold winter days and lunches lovingly packed in our lunch boxes. I remember laying on the kitchen floor, our feet in sandwich bags waving in the air so mom could shove our feet into boots assembly line-style before we went out to play. I remember her doing the dishes and laundry long after I was supposed to be in bed because she had spent the whole day with us. I remember crying my eyes out in frustration when I could not remember the 8's times tables and her doing them over and over and over again with me until I could do them—most of the time.

I remember sitting in the quiet stillness of the night; I remember piling on the bed as kids and later as grown-ups just to be with her. I remember her wearing a pig nose and eating chocolate cake gleefully on her birthday two days after surgery. I remember so many things, but mostly I remember her love. No matter where we were or what we were doing, she loved my dad, Katie, David, Liz, and me with out conditions, without bounds.

Even when she was serving others, which she did all the time, she tried to keep her focus on things that mattered to her family or things that would impact our lives too. When we were growing up, she was involved in what sometimes seemed like every activity known to man. She was a room mother in our classes, an avid high school sports fan, she helped lead our Brownie, Girl Scout, and Cub Scout troops. She knew all our teachers—by first name. She won the biggest award our school district gave, the Pillar of Parkway, recognizing her volunteerism and hours of service. She was involved in committee after committee after committee. She spearheaded something called Publishing House, where each student in our school wrote their own book and had it published in a binder. She learned to read and type Braille so the blind children in our school could be included. She went on field trips with us, and I think she had more fun than we did. One time on a field trip, she rescued one of Katie's friends out of a lake—not worried that she, too, would spend the rest of the day squelching around in wet tennis shoes. I am sure that she made Katie's friend feel like it was a great adventure going to visit the fishies instead of allowing her to feel foolish and embarrassed for falling in the lake in the first place. Mom could do that, make you feel good about bad situations, help you grow from them, learn from them, and change from them.

It is funny how sometimes parents turn everything into a lesson. Mom had that gift, but until recently never realized that she was a teacher. That was one of her goals almost as far back as I can remember, and she was always a little disappointed she never had the chance to go back and finish school. A few weeks ago, she and I were lying in the bed talking about her life and what was important to her. That day she realized that despite the fact that she never held a degree in her hand, she had been a teacher her whole life. She had achieved her goal after all. She taught many people valuable lessons about life and how to live. How to not just survive but thrive, how to serve with a smile and a grateful heart. How to wake up in the morning and praise God for giving her the gift of another day and how to make that day perfect. She was able to minister to those around her, guide people through pain and loss. She had an amazing capacity to see the goodness in people and help them realize and achieve their true potential. She was a living example of faith in action, of courage in spite of enormous obstacles and odds, of gratitude to the give of life and how to find true joy and peace in any situation.

Mom faced her illness with great courage and faith. She was an example and an inspiration. She touched many lives. So many people watched how she survived with cancer, and about two years ago, mom was asked to give a speech at the American Cancer Societies Survivor day. In part of her speech she said this, "God's answer to my frustration was clear. He showed me the strengths I had developed. I am doing what He wants with my life. I have grown; I have become stronger. I am doing the best I can do. I am not alone in this journey through life. I have grown more confident in the woman I now am and not the woman I dreamed I would be. I saw my worth when I understood that my experience could provide a source of strength and hope for other survivors. I have learned success in the doing, not the getting, the trying not the triumph. I have learned that joy is available to everyone, but you can not expect it to find you, sometimes you have to go look for it."

Joy, Faith, Hope, Courage, Love, Service, Strength, Gratitude— all of these words express some important aspect of my mother. Things that made her worthy of being the person I want to grow up to be like. For these things I am grateful.

My mom always enjoyed music. During her illness it comforted her. The last few months, some of my most precious times with her were spent singing or listening to music. Several months ago, my church choir sang a song that summarizes my mom well. As I close, I would like to share that song with you.

Faithful by Geron Davis—Song of Praise [2]

When others would have quit you kept on going
When someone stopped to rest you just pressed on
You never lost your passion or your vision
Always faithful to the Lord and to his song.

I know that there were times it wasn't easy
I'm sure you tasted failure once or twice
But that just never seemed to change your purpose
Or the calling that God placed upon your life.

<CHORUS>
You were faithful to through the hard times
Faithful through the night
Committed to the kingdom
And faithful to the fight
Faithful as a leader,

Faithful as a friend
I am grateful
You were faithful

The span of those you've touched can not be measured
The difference you made eternally
Until the book of all your deeds is open
revealed today for all the world to see

Then one by one they each will tell their story
recounting all you did along the way
And when today you stood before your leader
I know with out a doubt you heard him say

<CHORUS>
You were faithful to through the hard times
Faithful through the night
Committed to the kingdom
And faithful to the fight
Faithful as a leader,
Faithful as a friend
I am grateful
You were faithful

You were faithful

I know one of my mother's greatest wishes would be that her life and her example can help make you all faithful heroes.
Thank you.